Functional Movement Practice using Kettlebells

By

Uri Hirsch

Founder of Kettlebells Training in Israel

תרגול תנועתי תפקודי באמצעות קטלבלס

(Hebrew: Tirul Tnuati Tifkudi Im Kettlebells)

Written by: **Uri Hirsch**
Translated by: **Mike Garmise**
Illustrations by: **Olga Aharonov Koriansky**
Cover Design and Photography: **Chen Ziv, Zohar Ron**
Photography: **Marina Wasserman Samson**
Demonstrations by: **Rinat-ya Alon, Ron Oren**

First edition - 2013

Where the male gender appears in the book, this is only for convenience in writing and editing. The material is intended for men and women alike.

Functional-movement practice does not deal with the exerciser only at the physical level. This type of practice constitutes a part of one's life culture; it is an auxiliary tool for improving physical functioning and maintaining a healthy, balanced life style. The aim of the book is to encourage the culture of practice and movement, as part of one's physical culture.

TABLE OF CONTENTS

Introduction

"As long as a person exercises and works a lot and is not satisfied, and his intestines are loose - no sickness can come upon him and he will become stronger, even if he eats bad foods; he who sits comfortably and does not exercise... even if he eats good foods and maintains himself according to medical practice, all his days will be painful and his energies depleted" (Maimonides, Laws of Knowledge 4, 14-15).

In today's culture, "**exercising**" implicitly refers to engaging in physical fitness training. But it shouldn't. Rather it should refer to the general effort made by a body as part of physical work. Engaging in physical work requires us to activate and mobilize the entire body, as a result of which we will be healthier and therefore feel better too.

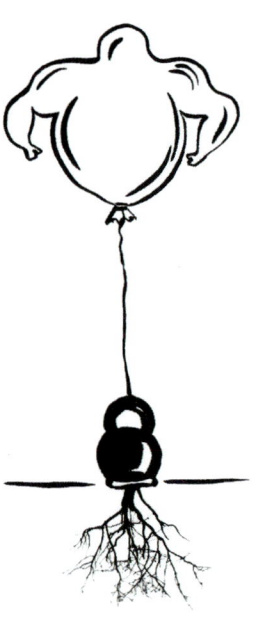

The material hedonism and technological progress that have become central elements in today's Western culture have essentially made body activation and movement unnecessary. To compensate, we set aside time for specific activities that will provide our bodies with what they need. Western training culture, like that in Ancient Greece, began with the desire to have a well-shaped physical appearance and evolved into an emphasis on nurturing the body as a supreme objective. In other words, the spirit was removed and the focus became physical. In Jewish culture (as in Eastern cultures), engaging in physical activity is a means of assisting us to maintain bodily health through awareness and an effort to build a deeper inner world.

There are free men whose spirit is that of a slave, and there are slaves whose spirit is full of freedom; one who is true to his own self - is truly a free man, and one whose whole life is only what is good and fair in the eyes of others - is a slave" (Rabbi Avraham Yitzhak Hacohen Kook)

Functional movement practice, as I see it, is about our ability to function better and more effectively in our daily lives, according to our individual needs.

The practice in this book diverts the emphasis from "how the body looks" to "how the body functions" and its corollary "how I feel."

Practice deals with acquiring movement skills with an emphasis on optimal technique and its consequent improvement in fitness components. It is important for each of us to be able to master and perform the basic movement components such as crawling, jumping, climbing, skipping, pulling, pushing, lunging, lifting, catching, throwing, moving and protecting ourselves. While moving quickly over long distances from one place to another, we should be able to lift and carry heavy objects, overcome obstacles, perform tasks accurately and with good timing, and respond to the environment and to unexpected situations. Meeting these demands requires several actions that can be implemented simultaneously with maximal efficiency and with as few injuries as possible. In a perfect world there would be no need to practice drills to improve strength, flexibility, endurance, coordination and speed...

> **The more the world develops, the more it strives to return to its original state"** (Rabbi Avraham Yitzhak Hacohen Kook)

In this book I have taken the liberty of straying somewhat from the usual terminology of the fitness world, replacing it with simple, clear language that can provide an auxiliary aid for instructors and exercisers. Teachers and instructors of movement and fitness must understand and explain that functional movement practice is not merely exercises or using new types of apparatus ("fitness toys"). Rather it is a systematic, long-range approach to practice, which includes the acquisition of extensive knowledge, logic and common sense that can serve as a useful tool in other practice and training systems as well.

Uri Hirsch, 2013

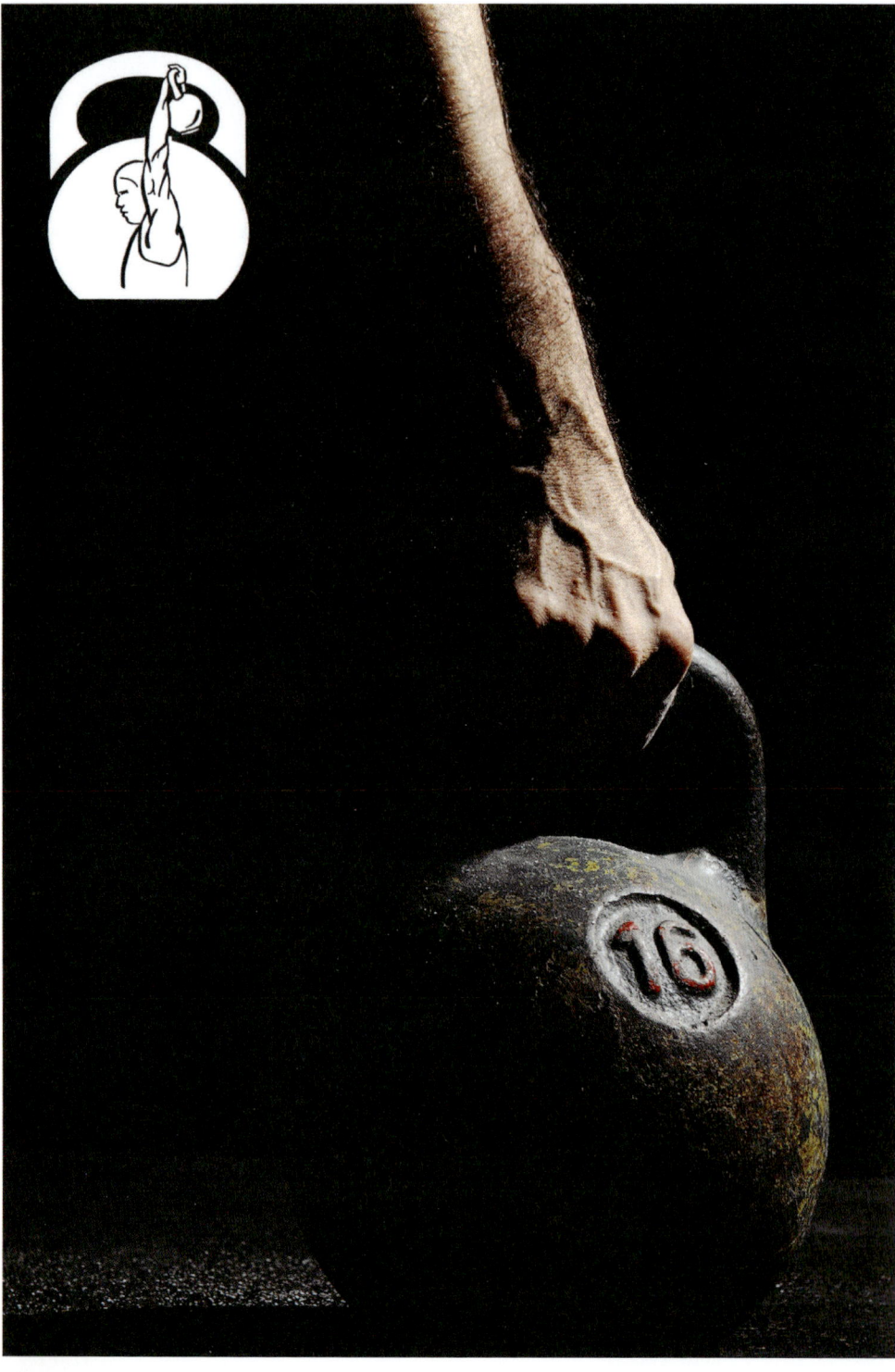

Chapter 1

Functional Movement Practice

- P–M–F

- Releasing our awareness

- The supreme goal of functional movement practice

- Practical objectives of functional movement practice

- The language of functional movement practice

- Basic movement patterns

1.1 P-M-F

When I think of physical activity, the picture that comes to mind is of activity that meets the basic needs of a healthy person. These include three components: Physical practice that focuses on our movement skills and abilities which enable us to improve our present and future functioning.

In short - PMF - Practice - Movement - Functioning

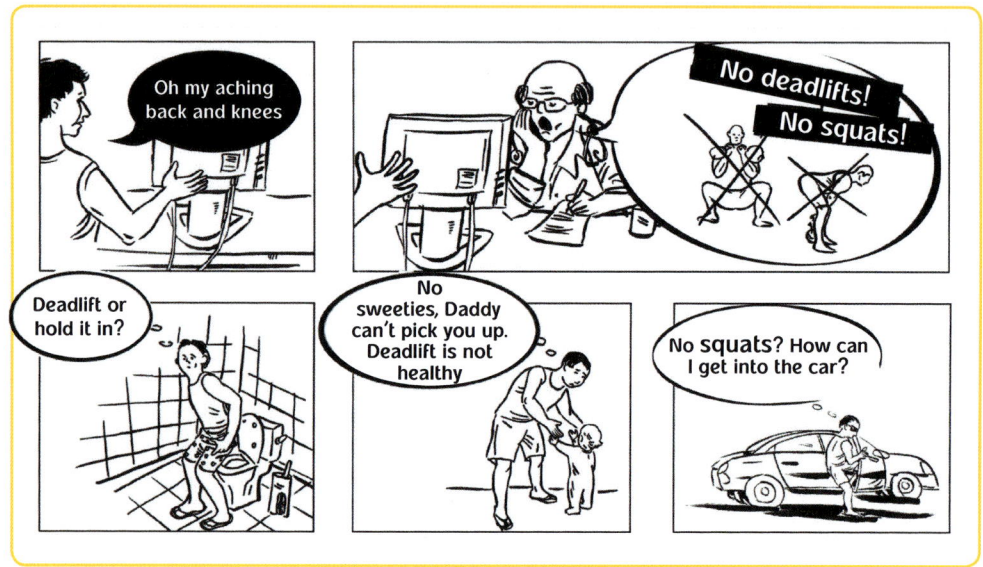

1.2 Releasing our awareness

Before we begin to work the body, it is important to understand the logic behind exercise and to free ourselves of certain commonly accepted assumptions. As I mentioned in the introduction, our physical culture changed from the aspiration to achieve a sculpted physical appearance to a view of body care as a supreme value. We are hostages to a worldview that has imprisoned our awareness and does not allow us to see that we are slaves to a materialistic culture, in a world whose reference point for almost all things is material. We have lost sight of the essence of our workouts (and lives) and have become addicted to the external form, the beautiful sculpted look that can be achieved through physical practice.

1.3 The supreme goal of functional movement practice

The basic aim in functional movement practice is to prepare our bodies and minds properly for the functional tasks that exercisers - and all others - must perform in daily life and in dealing with special tasks and conditions.

1.4 Practical objectives of functional movement practice

- Restoring and preserving our basic abilities and reducing potential damage in daily life (physical deterioration, sedentary life, excessive loads...)
- Learning and improving simple skills, mastering a broad array of movements, integrating movement patterns and creating a variety of neuronal patterns that form the automatic system (much like spoken vocabulary).
- Physical programming - combining and connecting complex skills, complex techniques, and movement sequences into one flow, and combining physical fitness components in a way that is adapted, coordinated and balanced for the individual exerciser.
- Creating a repertoire of skills and abilities to serve as "insurance" when encountering unexpected situations in the future and to slow down the functional decline associated with old age.

1.5 The language of functional movement practice

Movement practice vs. physical training - In physical training, the aim is to utilize intensive, challenging work to improve various fitness components. In movement practice the aim is to learn movements and skills and to internalize correct technique until it becomes automatic.

Mobility vs. muscles - The human body is required to perform a wide variety of tasks. For us to perform these tasks more effectively and to minimize injuries, we must drill the body in a way that improves its movement abilities and skills (mobility). **Why mobility?** Because the brain, which controls and activates our muscles through the nervous system, works and thinks in terms of fully coordinated movement and not in terms of contracting specific muscles. Because when we practice mobility instead of exercising individual muscle contractions, we evaluate exercises according to which movement I am performing and not according to which muscles I am activating. For example: **pushing while standing** involves activation of leg, core, chest, shoulder and arm muscles.

In daily life we do not stop and analyze which muscles we are using in a given action. We simple do what is appropriate, as we will see below.

Do you want to get up from the chair? Turn a page...? Forget about strengthening muscles - and begin to improve your mobility.

1.6 Basic movement patterns

Movement ability is composed of movement patterns. Our basic movement patterns are: squat, lift, lunge, twist, push, pull, walk and run. For the most part, basic movement patterns do not occur in isolation but rather in some integrated form.

Pattern	Uses
Squat	Rising from a sitting position, jumping
Lift	Lifting objects
Lunge	Clearing an obstacle, skipping

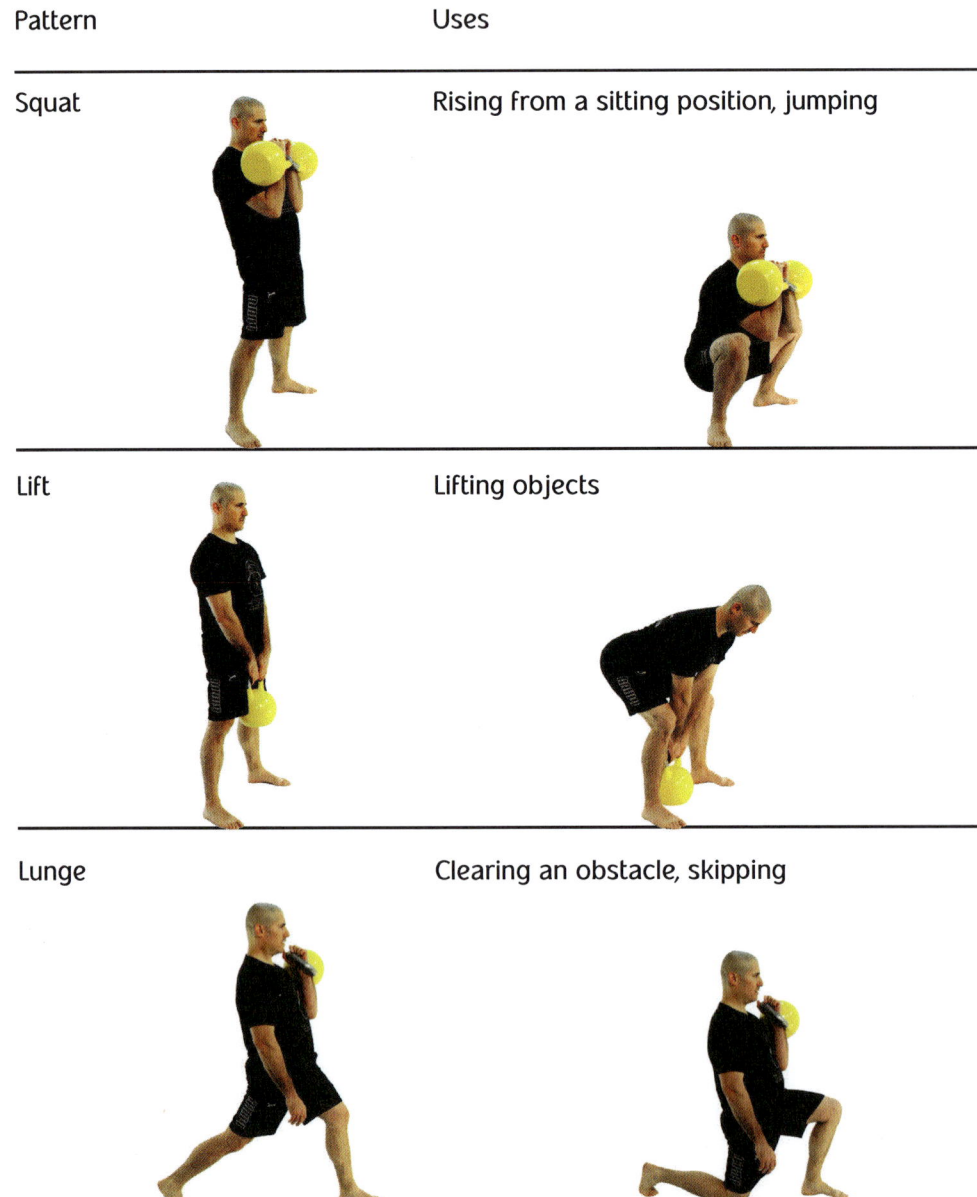

Twist

Integrated in throwing, climbing, crawling

Push

Throwing, punching

Pull

Climbing, towing, carrying

Walk

Walking, running

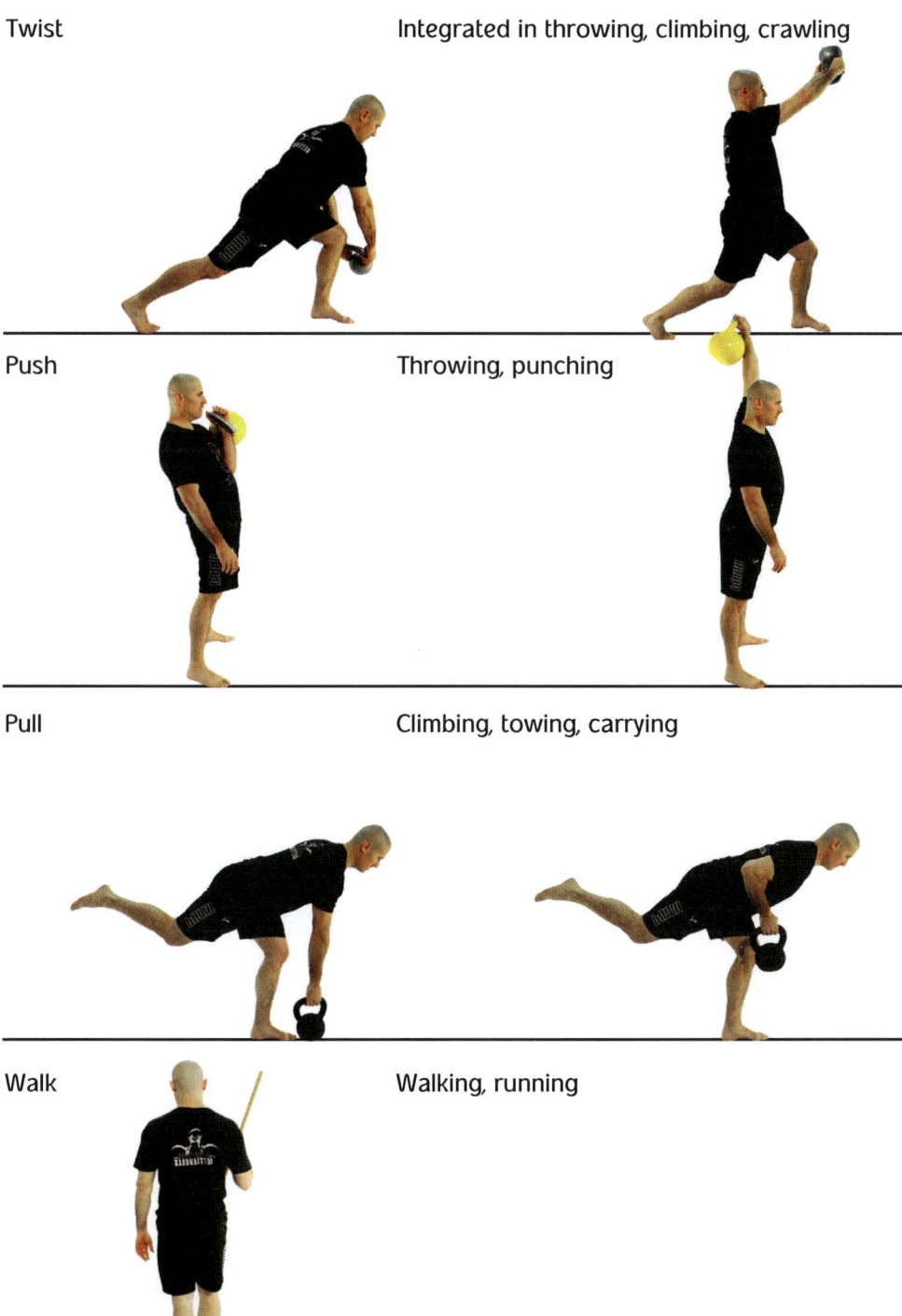

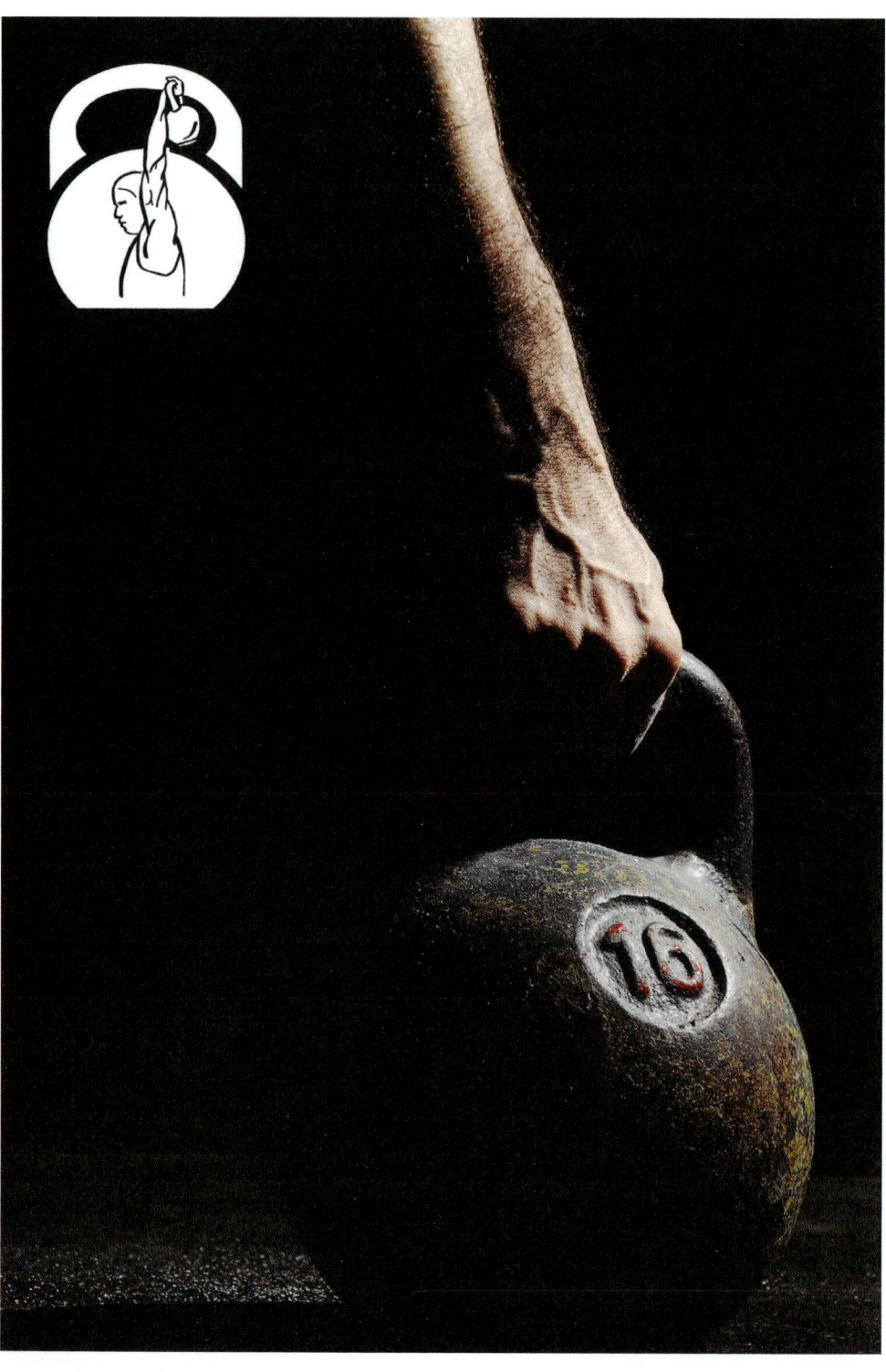

Chapter 2

Components of Functional Movement Practice

- Joint stability and mobility

- Balance and maintaining the center of gravity over the base of support

- Kinetic (movement) chains

- Physical fitness

- Motor implementation

- Comparative table: Functional movement practice vs. muscle training

How we function is affected by our mastery of physical abilities as well as by external factors that influence our body's ability to move. When examining each exercise in our practice program, it is important for us to recognize and understand these components. With proper understanding of the components we will better be able to select suitable exercises and also answer questions such as: What is the logic of choosing these exercises and how they are performed? Do they meet our needs?

2.1 Joint stability and mobility

The body is composed of a kinetic (movement) chain, a collection of joints beginning in the feet and ending at the head. Each joint may affect - and be affected by - the joint below and/or above it. Each joint and chain of joints has a designated function. Each joint should be exercised according to its needs, so that it can function freely and optimally.

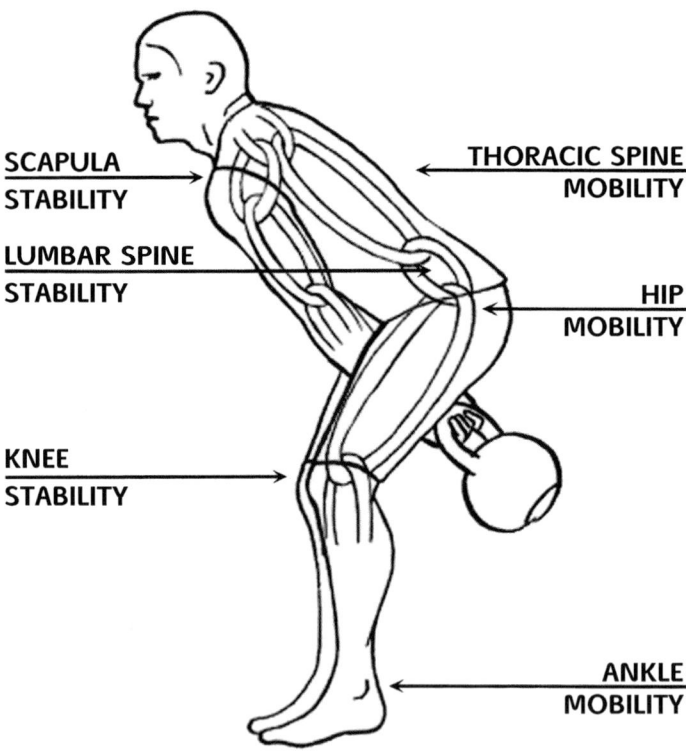

SCAPULA STABILITY

THORACIC SPINE MOBILITY

LUMBAR SPINE STABILITY

HIP MOBILITY

KNEE STABILITY

ANKLE MOBILITY

Before beginning to exercise joints or muscles, we must define what the joints need. First, however, we must differentiate between:

Joint stability - the ability to control movement in a joint (control of excess movement or fixation of a limb).

Joint Mobility - the ability to produce full movement with the joint.

JOINT	FUNCTION	FAULTY FUNCTIONING
Wrist	Movement	
Elbow	Stabilization	
Shoulder/arm	Movement	
Scapula	Stabilization	
Thoracic spine	Movement	Lack of mobility in the thoracic spine may cause excessive movement in the cervical or lumbar spine (which is supposed to stabilize and not move)
Lumbar spine	Stabilization	
Pelvis/hip	Movement	Lack of movement in the hip may cause excessive movement in the knee or lumbar spine (which are supposed to stabilize and not move)
Knee	Stabilization	
Ankle	Movement	Lack of movement in the ankle may cause excessive movement in the knee (which is supposed to stabilize and not move)
Foot	Stabilization	

Table 1: Joint stability and mobility

Movement compensation
A direct connection can be found between injuries/pain and improper/lack of joint functioning. Lack of functioning (loss of mobility or of stability) in a given joint may cause movement compensation in the adjacent joint, which we may experience as pain in that joint or another joint in the kinetic (movement) chain.

Examples of improper chain movement and its consequences:
The most common example the consequences of improper movement can be found in the lower back. The lumbar spine is supposed to provide stability. But lack of mobility in the pelvis/hip (the joint under the spine) may cause compensatory movement by the lumbar spine (which is supposed to provide stabilization and not movement).

Other examples:
- Lack of ankle mobility may lead to knee pain.
- Lack of pelvic/hip mobility may cause lower back or knee pain.
- Lack of thoracic spine mobility may lead to pain in the shoulder girdle, neck or lower back.

When practicing it is necessary to relate to all body joints according to functional needs. It is essential to mobilize and soften the ranges of movement for joints that are supposed to be mobile and to strengthen (without stiffening) the joints required for stability.

Stability of the lumbar spine (Core stability)
The lumbar spine is supposed to be stable (the opposite of mobile) and to maintain its stability under all loads no matter how unusual or unexpected.

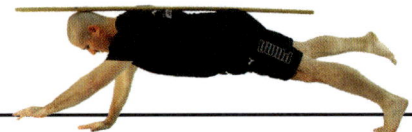

Spinal stability is achieved by strengthening and arching (without drawing in) the trunk* – creating a type of muscle band that increases lumbar spine stability and enables it to withstand high loads.

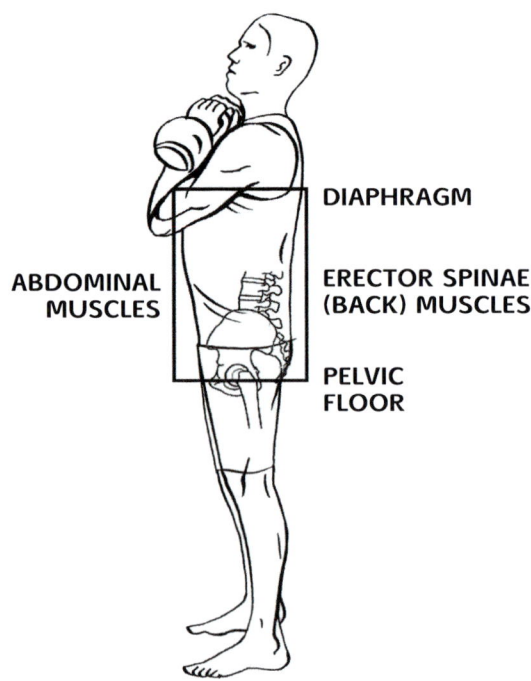

DIAPHRAGM

ABDOMINAL
MUSCLES

ERECTOR SPINAE
(BACK) MUSCLES

PELVIC
FLOOR

***The trunk** is the central part of the body. It includes the back and spine, buttocks, abdomen and chest. The upper end of the trunk is delineated by the shoulder girdle and the lower end is marked by the pelvic girdle.

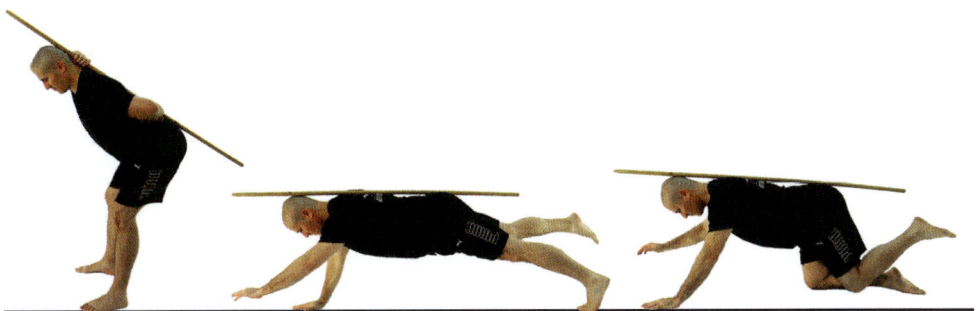

The process of developing lumbar spine stability – from isolating the core muscles to controlled coordination of complex movement

Something to think about:
If we understand the idea and importance of lumbar spine stability, why do we practice mobility of the lumbar spine (in various types of sit-ups)?

Why do we practice lumbar spine stability in isolation?
Isolating and activating a specific muscle or fitness component contradicts our approach to practice. Nevertheless, we isolate muscle groups in a number of cases:

- When we progress from isolation to integration and from simple to complex
- In order to create awareness of spinal stability
- When it is necessary to strengthen the weak "link" in the kinetic chain

After isolated practice we return to the whole complex movement, in order to test the exerciser's ability to implement what was practiced – to stabilize the body in a given movement task.

2.2 Balance and keeping the center of gravity above the base of support

The ability to maintain balance and to keep our center of gravity above its base of support is an important component of functionality, from the basic level of moving the body (walking, overcoming obstacles), to applying power in order to move or prevent movement imposed by external resistance (pushing and pulling), in a static position (standing on one leg) or in movement (skipping). Proprioceptors supply the body with information about our balance and the location of our limbs in the space around us and where our body parts are during movement (without our actually looking at them). They also help us to regulate the energy and speed we expend against external resistance.

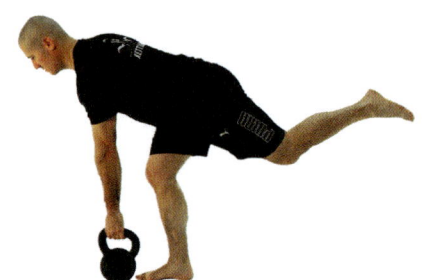

2.3 Kinetic (movement) chains

In our daily lives, our lower limbs work more in closed kinetic chain patterns (squatting, lifting), while our upper limbs work for the most part in open kinetic chain patterns (pushing, pulling). Actual functioning requires the integration and coordination of closed and open kinetic chains.

Closed kinetic chain – A movement pattern in which the end of the limb in movement is not free to move and a predictable chain movement is created from that joint to other joints in the kinetic chain.

For example, when squatting, the foot is fixed on the floor and creates a coordinated movement of the other joints above the foot - the ankle, knee and hip.

Open kinetic chain - A movement pattern in which the end of the limb in movement is free to move and able to perform an isolated movement without involving movement in the other joints.

For example, in leg extension apparatus, the foot is free to move and it is possible to move the knee without moving the ankle or hip.

As I mentioned above, the body is a kinetic chain, a collection of joints that extends from the feet to the head. While each joint has its own designated function, a chain connection links groups of joints as a whole.

Types of kinetic chains:

1. Posterior chain
Function: Extension and hyperextension of the spine (as well as flexion of the knee and extension of the ankle).
Components: The posterior of the body - foot, ankle, lower leg, knee, thigh, spine.
Illustrative exercise: Good morning

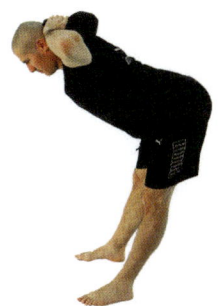

2. Anterior chain
Function: Flexion of the spine and hip (as well as extension of the knee and flexion of the ankle).
Components: The anterior of the body - top of foot, lower leg, knee, thigh, pelvis, abdomen, ribs, chest.
Illustrative exercise: Get-up stage 2 - from supine to elbow

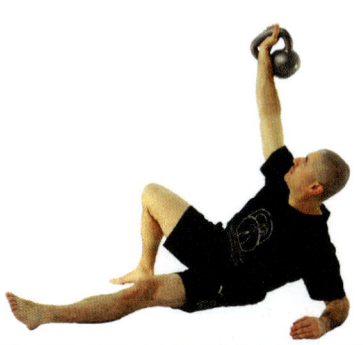

3. Lateral chain

Function: Side flexion of the spine, abduction of the hip and external rotation of the ankle.

Components: The external part of the body - lateral side of the foot, lower leg, knee, thigh, pelvis, oblique abdominals, ribs.

Illustrative exercise: Windmill

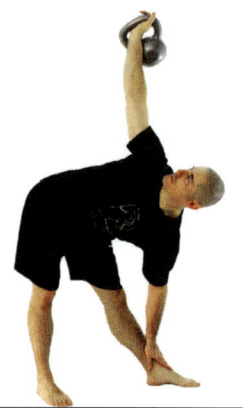

4. Rotational chain

Function: Rotational movement in the spine and simultaneous stabilization of the spine and legs.

Components: The posterior and anterior of the body - back of skull, cervical spine, scapulae, lateral ribs, anterior pelvis, anterior lateral knee, heel, posterior lateral knee, sitting bones, coccyx, spine, posterior of skull.

Illustrative exercise: Wood chop

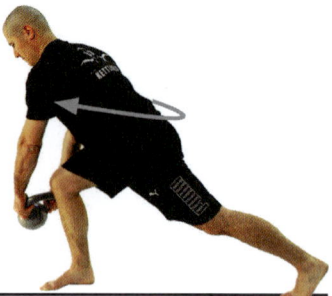

5.1 Shoulder-arm chain - Pulling
Function: Pull an object toward the body and stabilize our body while leaning back on the hands.
Components: The posterior of the body - thoracic and cervical (chest and neck) vertebrae, scapulae, arm, forearm to fingertips.
Illustrative exercise: 1 L Dead-lift + pull

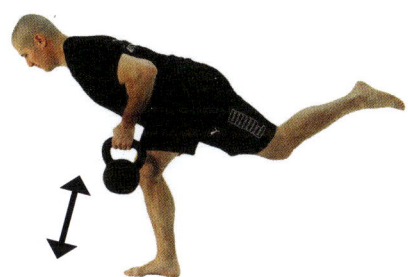

5.2 Shoulder-arm chain - pushing
Function: Push an object from the body and stabilize our body while leaning forward on our hands.
Components: The anterior of the body - upper ribs, chest, shoulder, arm, forearm to fingertips.
Illustrative exercise: push ups

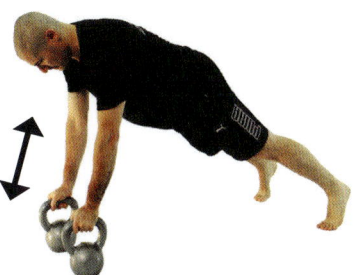

6.1 Functional chain – posterior
Function: Connect the lower and upper parts of the body and provide more power and accuracy to the limbs.
Components: The anterior of the body - from the upper external end of the tibia to the buttocks and on a diagonal line through the latissimus dorsi to the upper end of the humerus (arm bone).
Illustrative exercise: 1 L Dead-lift

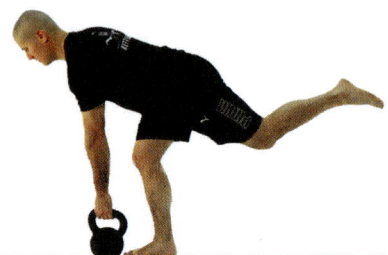

6.2 Functional chain – anterior
Components: The anterior of the body - front of the thigh, on a diagonal line through the external part of the abdomen and chest to the upper end of the humerus (arm bone).
Illustrative exercise: Get-up Stage 2 - from supine to elbow

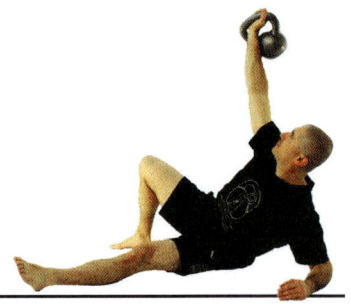

Kinetic chains
The body functions by integrating many muscle groups (and connective tissues) that work in coordination. These create kinetic chains. Understanding the kinetic chains and our movement patterns enables us to form a better idea of how our body functions, and what we can expect and demand of it in practice. It can also be used as a tool for identifying kinetic limitations - and removing them by improving our mobility.

2.4 Physical fitness

Physical fitness refers to the entire array of abilities a human develops for performing physical actions, from daily tasks to complex athletic performance. Connecting and integrating all of the physical fitness components into one set is an essential precondition for improving functioning. However, fitness is not an end in itself - we do not need to be the strongest woman on the block and strength has no meaning if we do not have the ability to use it. We do not need to be the most flexible guy around - flexibility is meaningless if we cannot use it to create movement. We do not have to be the most... (choose your fitness component); such a component is meaningless if we do not have the ability to (choose your implementation). Physical fitness enables us to be mobile and gives us the ability to crawl, jump, climb, skip, pull, push, lunge, lift, catch, throw, move and protect ourselves. In other words, functional movement practice improves all of our physical and cognitive fitness components as a whole.

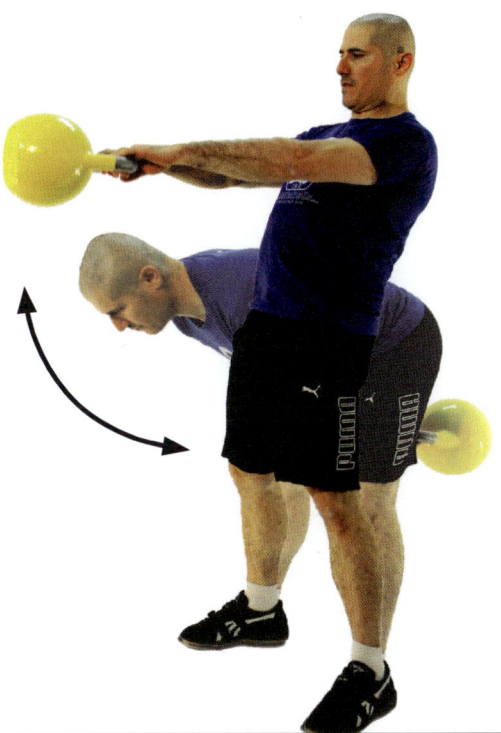

COMPONENT	DEFINITION	EXAMPLE
Endurance	The ability to continue to perform actions over a period of time	The ability to continue lifting kettlebells time and again
Flexibility	The ability to perform movements in the optimal range of joint movement, without compensation by adjacent joints	Lack of flexibility in the pelvis/hip causes movement compensation in the spine
Strength / Explosive power	The ability to activate maximal strength in a fast movement	To overcome body and kettlebell weight in as little time as possible
Power	The ability to overcome external resistance	To overcome body and kettlebell weight
Speed	The ability to perform a movement in as little time as possible	Accelerating the body and the kettlebells
Coordination	The ability to coordinate movement components and create movement balance	Coordination and timing of joint movements during deadlift
Agility	The ability to change body position and movement direction quickly and accurately	Shifting kettlebells from hand to hand
Regulation of strength	The ability to regulate strength level to create movement that is accurate and without tension or stiffness in body parts that do not contribute to the movement	Activating balanced strength to resistance and moving the pelvis forward while at the same time relaxing the arms and shoulders
Balance	The ability of the body to maintain equilibrium	Maintaining the center of gravity above the base of support during deadlift

Proprioception	Sensing the location of body parts. The system of unconscious internal receptors for posture and movement	Sensing the location of the spine during deadlift
Kinesthesis	The sensation of movement. Conscious sensation, without seeing body position	Sensing the location and distribution of body weight on the feet

Table 2: Physical Fitness Components

2.5 Motor implementation

As mentioned before, the brain works according to movement patterns. Therefore, functional movement practice includes the performance of a wide range of movement patterns that contain the positive transfer of ability and mobility components required for daily human needs as well as special skills.

There must be a connection between what we practice and what a task requires of us. On the one hand, an optimal environment must be created for learning and correcting improper movement patterns and internalizing optimal movement patterns. On the other hand, it is necessary to create varied and challenging activities that will produce a movement skill that can be internalized as an automatic response. In this way, when we resume performance of the required task, we will perform it better and more efficiently.

For example: Functional movement practice for the martial arts requires a broad range of motor abilities - balance, accuracy, timing, regulation of strength, force, agility, spatial orientation - in order to ensure a positive transfer to the special motor skills of jumping, throwing, kicking...

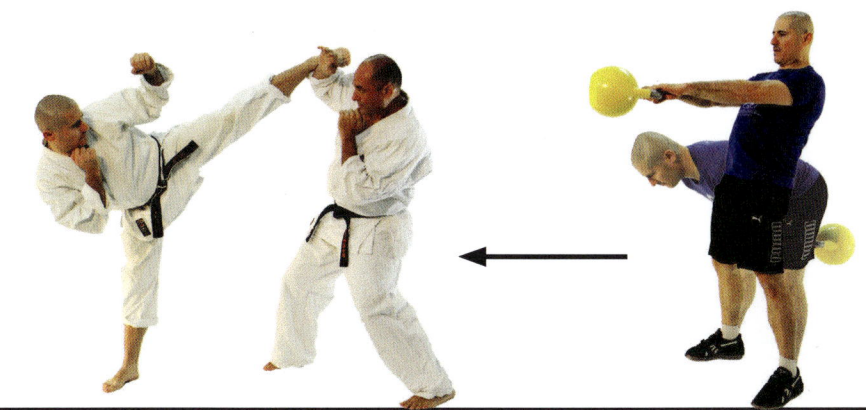

The bottom line is that functional movement practice is not a random collection of exercises. It is a systematic method of practice intended to attain defined aims. It is necessary to understand how the body functions so that we can identify the logic of posture and stability as well as the weaknesses and strong points of our movement, and to remove factors that limit the exerciser's movement (the main part of practice may be devoted to removing limiting factors and not to practicing special movement patterns). In other words, there must be logic in the order and choice of exercises.

2.6 Comparative table: Functional movement practice and muscle training

Muscle training usually concentrates on strengthening an individual muscle or muscle group in order to improve a specific fitness component in isolation from movement ability and with little consideration of the various components that may affect an exerciser's functioning. In contrast, the functional movement practice approach perceives the body as a unity of systems working in coordination where the connections and interactions linking body, thoughts and soul are of crucial importance.

	FUNCTIONAL MOVEMENT PRACTICE	MUSCLE TRAINING
Focus	Movement ability	Strengthening muscles
Exercises	Multi-joint	Isolated
Movement planes	Three-dimensional	Usually in the sagittal plane
Kinetic chain	Open and closed	Open
Exercise positions	Standing	Sitting/supine
Basic area and center of gravity	Integrated	
Movements	Authentic, from life (Squat)	Artificial/Apparatus (Knee extension on a machine)
Core muscles	Integrated	Separate exercises
Awareness and concentration	Integrated	Not required

Table 3: Comparison of functional movement practice and muscle training

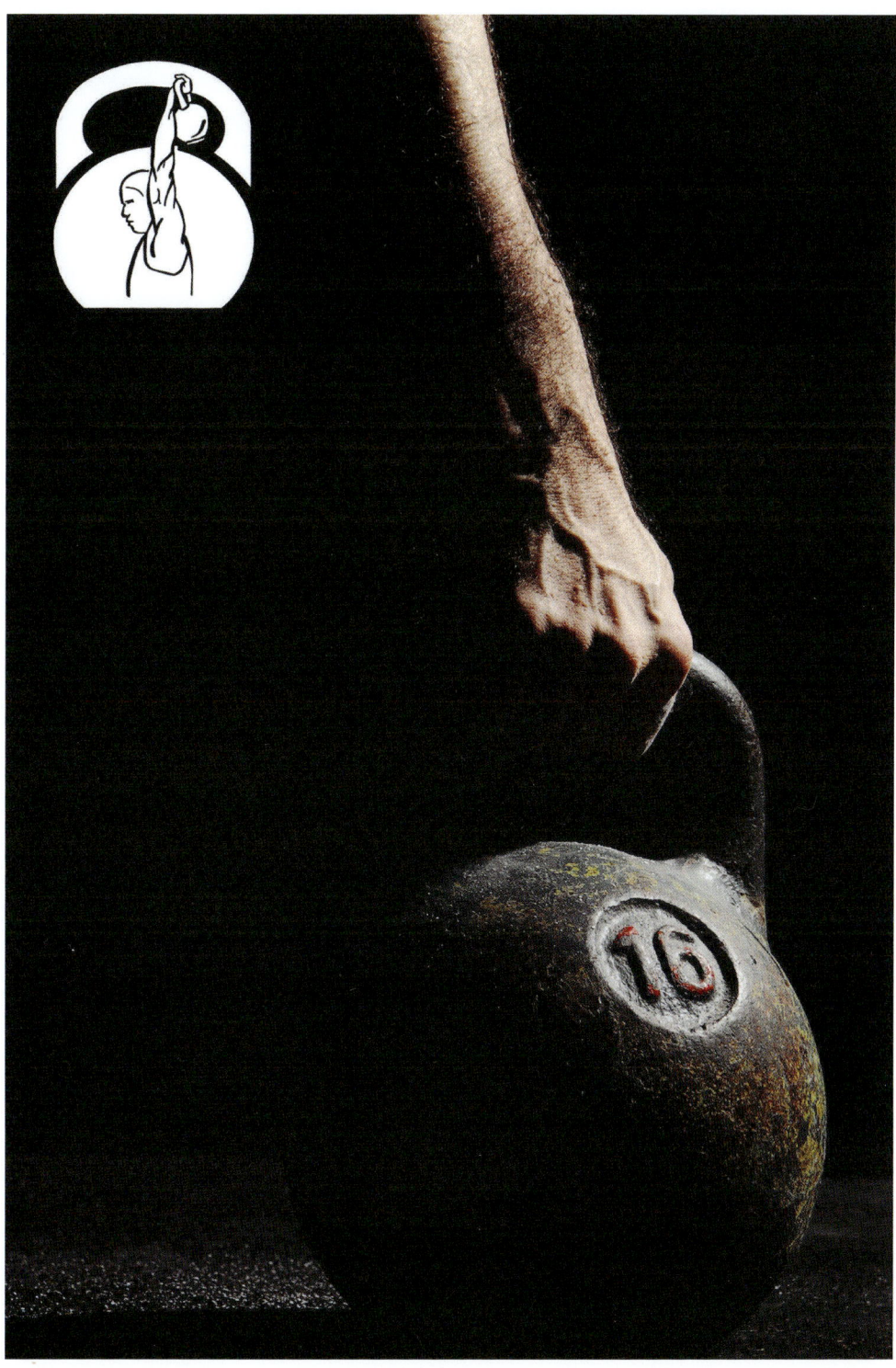

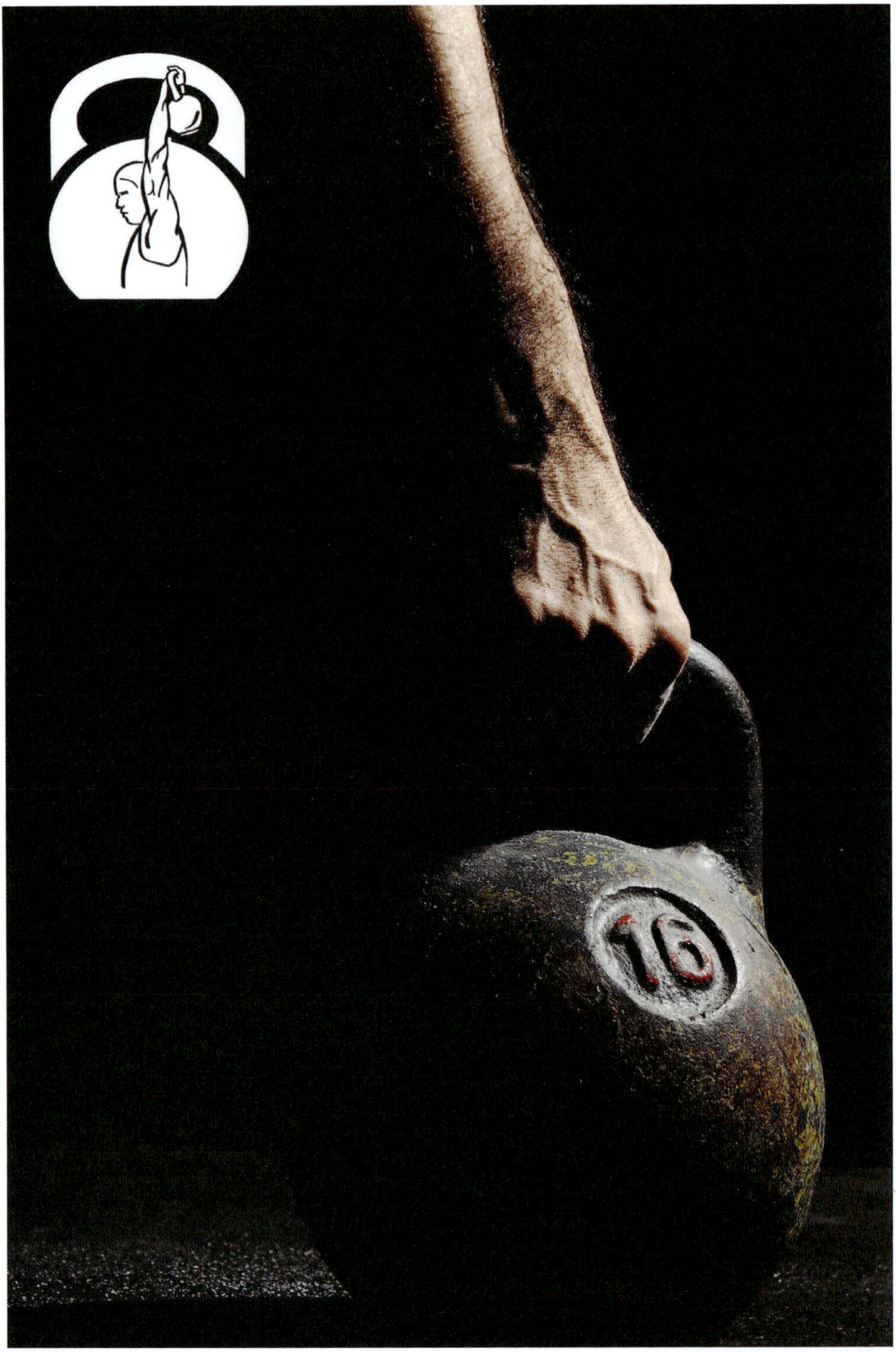

Chapter 3

Functional Movement Practice Using Kettlebells

- What is functional movement practice using kettlebells?

- The logic behind functional movement practice using kettlebells

- Kettlebells - Approaches and methods

3.1 What is functional movement practice using kettlebells?

Functional movement practice using kettlebells is based mainly on swings, on multi-joint movement that requires a high level of inter-joint coordination and high energetic expenditure. Practice is composed of exercises that improve movement ability and skills, and physical fitness components (power, strength, endurance, flexibility, speed, coordination, agility, balance, accuracy, reaction time) and as in life, practice using kettlebells also integrates several physical fitness components.

Through practice, the body learns to function as a whole coordinated unit with proper inter-limb timing: through the brain and nervous system the message is transmitted to muscles that provide the power to move the body - several different muscles are required for performing each exercise. Some are mobilizing muscles (which create movement in the joints that are supposed to move) and some are stabilizing muscles (which prevent movement in joints that are not supposed to move and on which force is applied to try to make them move).

The dynamics and flow of functional movement practice consume considerable energy. Such practice involves more muscle groups and combines both physical and cognitive elements (concentration, accuracy, coordination, balance and others). Exercisers learn how to perform daily movements more correctly and more efficiently, such as how to lift things from the floor and put them down, etc.

One of the great advantages of functional movement practice using kettlebells is that in a given period of time, practice improves a large number of physical abilities. It combines accuracy with flow, as in yoga; strength and force, as in weight lifting and martial arts; and energetic expenditure as in running.

3.2 The logic behind functional movement practice using kettlebells

The essence of practice using kettlebells is determined by their unique structure. Unlike regular weights, kettlebells are not balanced. The ball is far from the handle, which changes the kettlebells' center of gravity, and during practice the exerciser's center of gravity is moved out of equilibrium.

Kettlebell practice usually uses swinging motions - swinging the kettlebells transfers movement to all parts of the body, which must maintain its equilibrium and control and at the same time respond to the kettlebell movements. This ability is acquired through practice that dynamically engages the entire body.

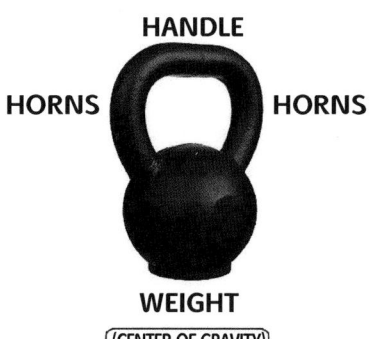

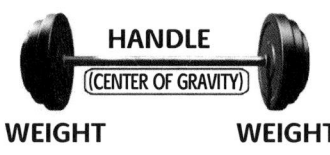

As in the martial arts, kettlebells also have a cycle of acceleration, effort and relaxation. The structure of the kettlebells allows us to relax the body between each effort. These "rest periods" enable us to practice at high intensity and for extended periods of time.

3.3 Kettlebells – Approaches and methods

There are two main approaches to kettlebell practice: kettlebells for fitness - and kettlebell swinging sport. The differences between the styles become evident from the defined aims and principles of each method. It is important to note that both styles require athletic ability and high technical skill but each style has its own special emphases and points of reference for performing the exercises.

Kettlebells for fitness

The fitness style of kettlebell practice is suited to the motivation shared by most exercisers - the desire to improve fitness components, improve posture, stimulate metabolism in order to lose weight, etc. This style, also called the hard style, is influenced by the martial arts and in fact incorporates some of their principles (such as Kime), and for that reason is also more widespread among martial arts devotees. Swings use aggressive whiplike movements, like sending a punch or kick.

In this style the whole body is mobilized for stability. Effort comes from the shoulder girdle and scapulae (shoulder blades), and swings are sharp, like sudden blows, in order to create the explosive power needed for moving the kettlebells. The style is somewhat similar to weight lifting or the explosive power of martial arts, and is suited mainly to high loads for relatively short periods. This style emphasizes variety - a broad range of exercises in supine or standing positions that are performed at various speeds, explosively and also slowly. The exercises characteristic of this style are get up, dead lift, squat, windmill and clean and press.

Kettlebell swinging as sport

Kettlebell swinging is a competitive sport activity, whose aim is to swing or jerk 32kg kettlebells as many times as possible within a 10 minute period.

Kettlebell lifting competitions are divided into two types:

Biathlon - composed of jerk and snatch

Long cycle - composed of clean and jerk.

This approach is also called the soft style. In this style the movement is soft, coordinated and flowing, like dance. The body learns to work freely for long periods of time, at high intensity, wasting as little energy as possible.

This style is based on efficiency, maximal accuracy, simplicity and economy of movement, so that competitors can continue to swing the required weight in the designated time for as many repetitions as possible.

Because we all differ in terms of our skeletal structure, genetics and other variables, reaching optimal performance requires adapting the swing to the exerciser's individual body build. To do this requires learning skills and high-level understanding by the coach and the exerciser. The three main exercises typical of this style are jerk, snatch and the long cycle, as well as auxiliary exercises.

Another style of kettlebell work is **juggling** -artistic kettlebell movement as part of performances or competitions. Kettlebell juggling is a free movement creation lasting about five minutes, in which the swinger presents an artistic segment composed of a sequence of complex swinging exercises at various levels of difficulty. Kettlebell juggling entails a much higher level of complexity and coordination than the first two styles and therefore, kettlebell jugglers must have appropriate training and high level skill.

In my opinion, as in the martial arts, it is impossible to determine which approach is best or most correct (assuming that the teacher is good). The suitability of the approaches or styles lies in the aims set by each exerciser. For this reason I have chosen to take the best from each style and to combine the components into a practice style suited to a broad cross section of exercisers, from amateurs to competitive athletes. Each one can adopt kettlebell exercises as a part of life, and each one can include personal emphases that will lead to optimal results using this method.

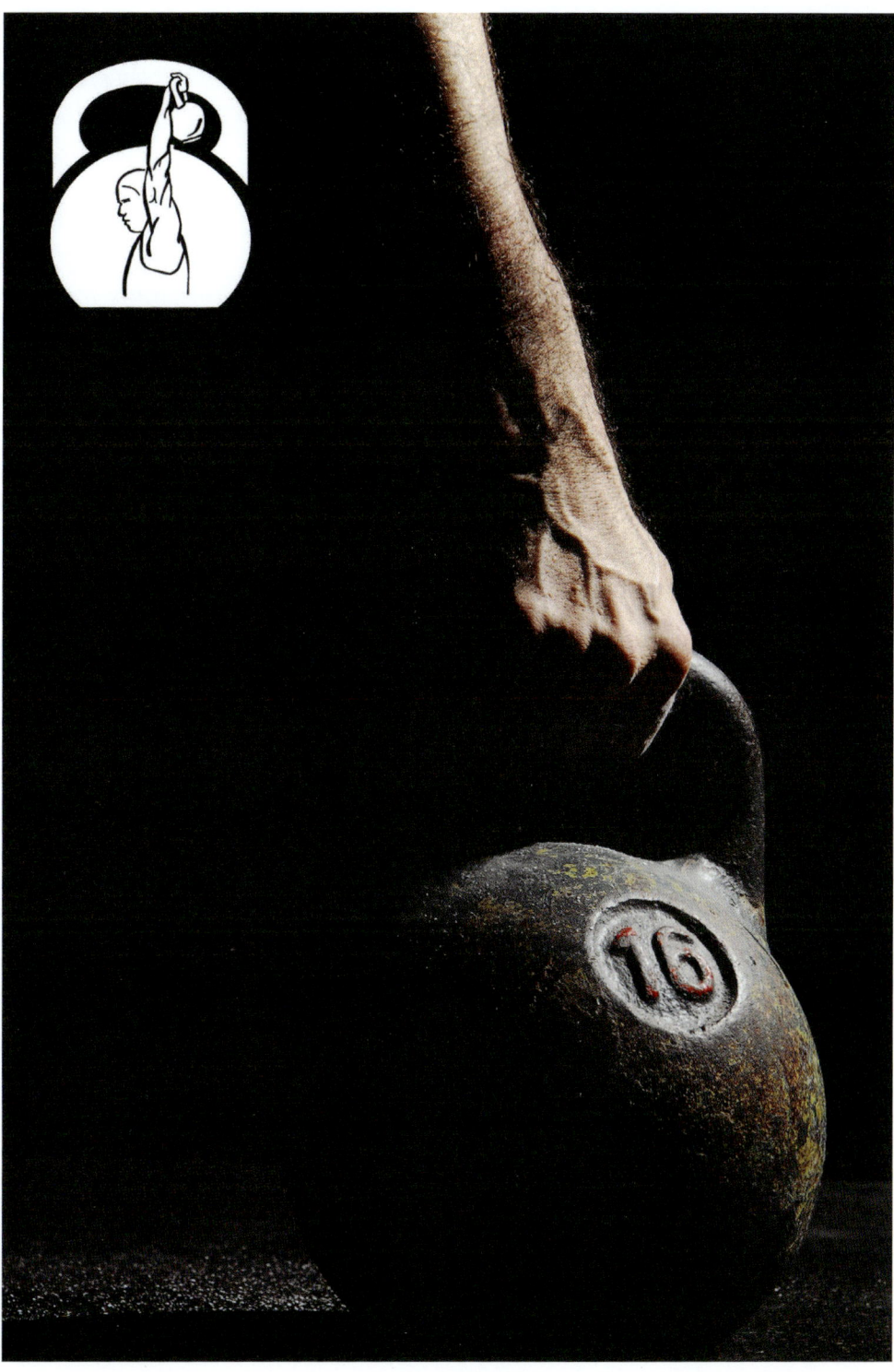

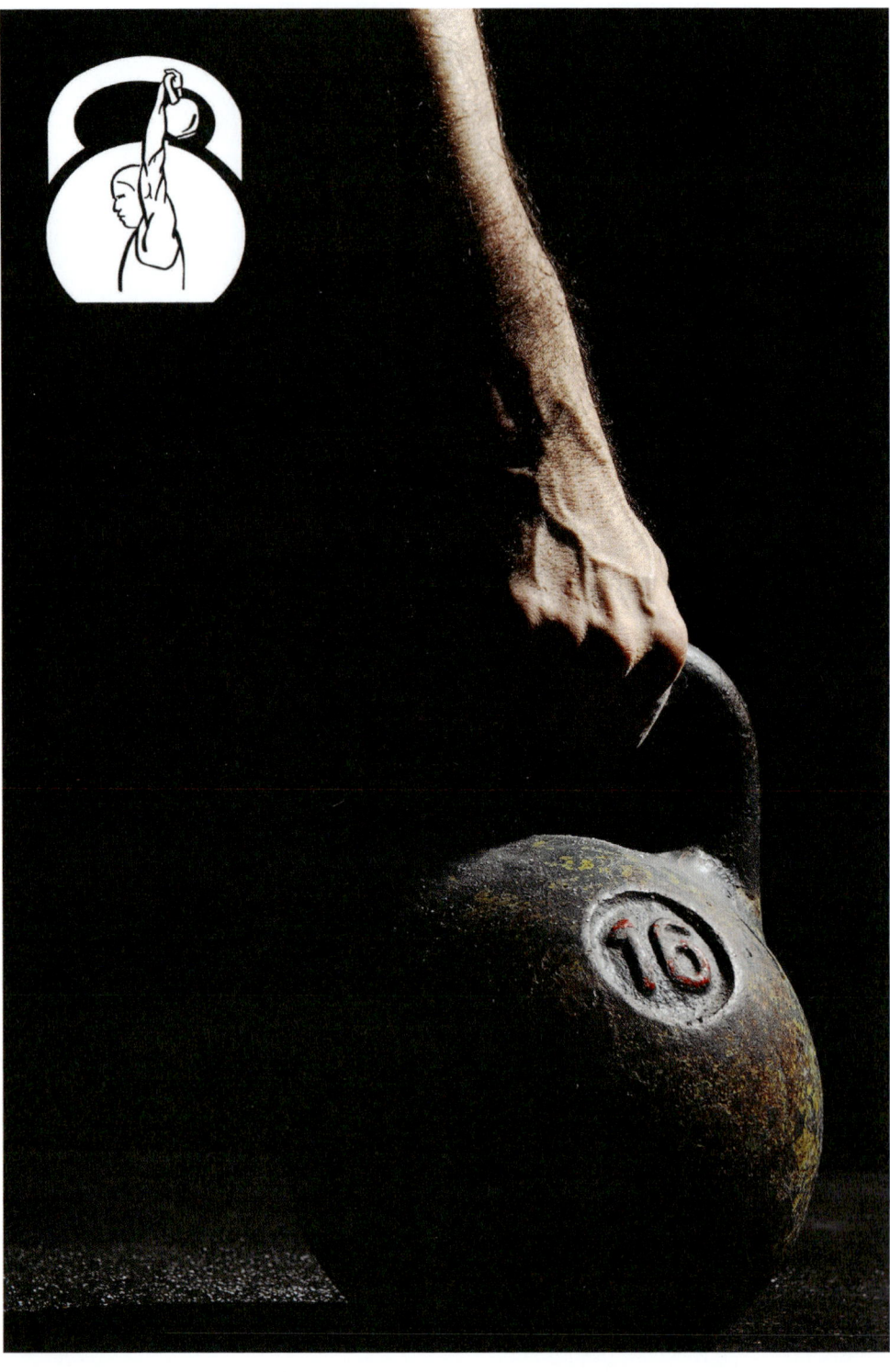

Chapter 4

From Theory to Practice

- Rating practice exercises

- Preparatory and release exercises

- Using high density foam rollers to release mobility limitations

- Mobility warm-up

- Practicing basic movement patterns

- Kettlebell exercises

4. From Theory to Practice

4.1 Rating practice exercises
- Pre-movement softening
- Mobility warm-up
- Practicing basic movement patterns
- Learning or improving technique
- Main exercise
- Moderate movement practice

4.2 Preparatory and release exercises
Preparing for practice - Mobility warm-up is intended to improve range of movement (using relaxation instead of stretches), remove factors that limit movement, and increase awareness.

Concluding the practice - Mobility exercise on high density foam rollers helps to relieve delayed muscle pains. Moderate mobility exercises gradually calm the body.

4.3 Using high density foam rollers to relieve mobility limitations
Connective tissue runs throughout our bodies, from head to toe, front and back. This tissue can be found around muscles, bones, ligaments, nerves and other internal organs. Its function is to maintain structural stability, protect, support and serve as a shock absorber.

Improper posture, limited movement, hypo- or hyper-activity and trauma can all cause movement limitations, which become a kind of "knot" in the connective tissue, leading to pain and limiting our ability to move. Through preliminary practice on a foam roller (rolling on it and applying pressure) we release these knots in the connective tissue, reduce stiffness and in this way improve the range and quality of movement.

Using the roller:
- Keeping the body limp, slowly roll on the roller, coordinating movements with breathing.
- Repeat 30-60 seconds on each side.
- 3 sets on each side
- Stop, hold a position and breathe while relaxing in especially stiff areas.

1 Thoracic spine
Hands support the head, buttocks in the air. Roll forward and backward over the rib cage area (from shoulders to solar plexus)

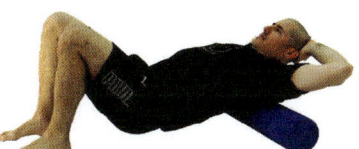

2 Shoulder blades (scapulae)
Hands support the head, elbows closed and buttocks in the air Roll forward and backward over the scapular (shoulder blade) area

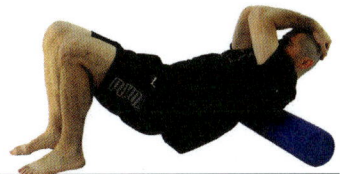

3 Latissimus dorsi and arm
Arms straight above head and buttocks in the air. Roll forward and backward over the armpit area (from arm to latissimus dorsi)

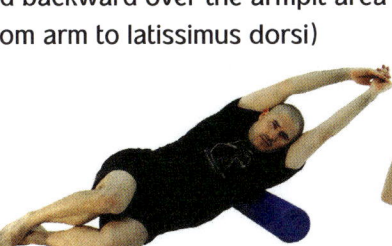

4 Twisting movement in the thoracic spine

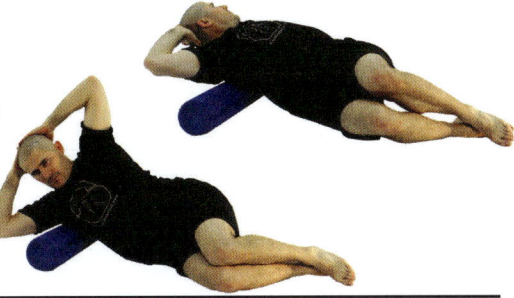

5 External (lateral) side of the hip
Roll forward and backward over the hip area (from pelvis to knee)

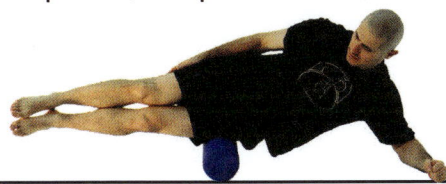

6 Front of thigh
Roll forward and backward over the thigh area (from pelvis to knee)

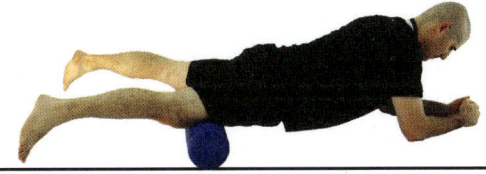

7 Calf (lower leg)
Roll forward and backward over the calf area (from knee to ankle)

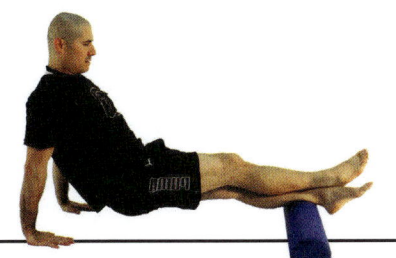

8 Buttocks
Roll forward and backward over the buttocks area (from pelvis to knee)

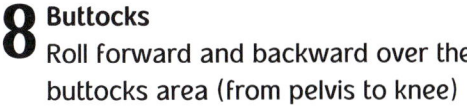
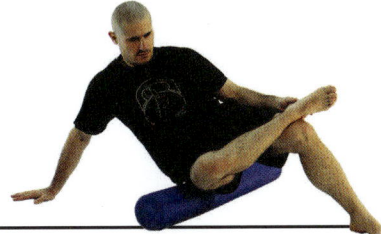

4.4 Mobility warm-up

We prepare the body for effort through a series of movements and positions performed in coordination with our breathing. The aim is to mobilize the joints, organize the body, remove factors that limit mobility and intensify our level of awareness as we prepare the body for exercise. One round is composed of two sets (right and left).

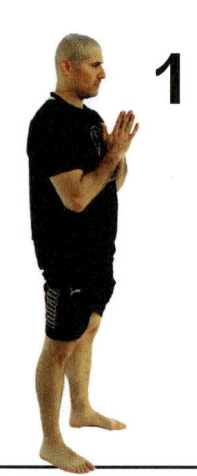

1

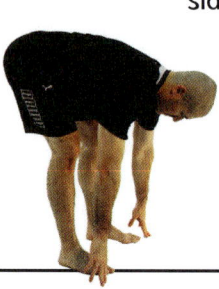

2 Raise arms while inhaling, and while exhaling, reach higher and back

3 While inhaling the sitting bones lengthen to the rear and while exhaling arms go down at the sides of the legs.

4 While inhaling the chest opens upward and the left leg moves to the rear

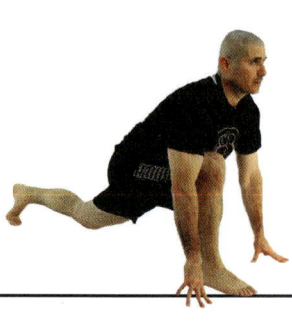

5 While inhaling the right arm opens

6 While holding the breath, the right arm returns and the right leg joins the left

7 While exhaling enter the supine position

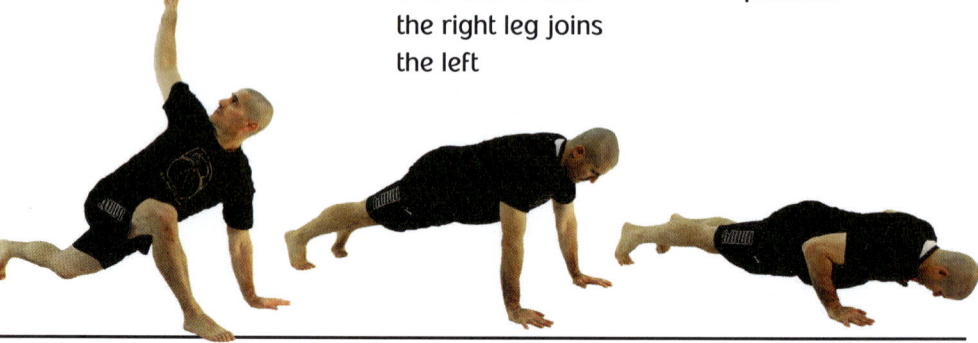

8 While inhaling the chest rises

9 While exhaling the pelvis rises and the chest pushes back and down

10 While inhaling the left leg goes up

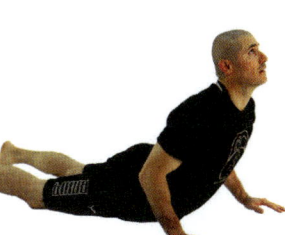
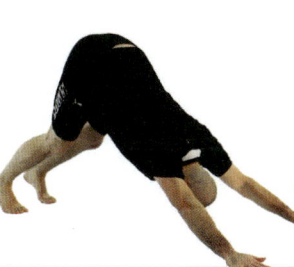
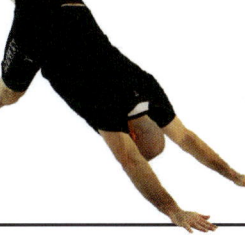

11 While exhaling the left leg returns to the position between the hands

12 While exhaling the body is bent over the left leg, right leg in the air

13 While exhaling the right leg joins the left one

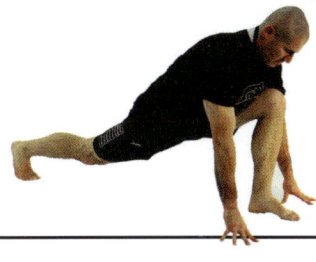
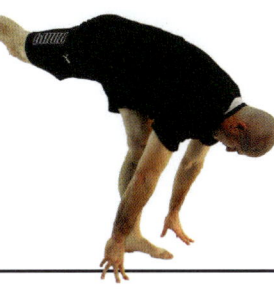
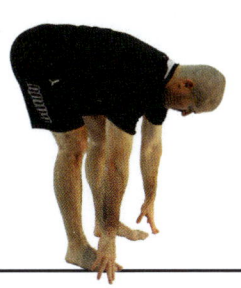

14 While inhaling the chest opens upward, arms are raised upward

15

16 Exhale and lower arms

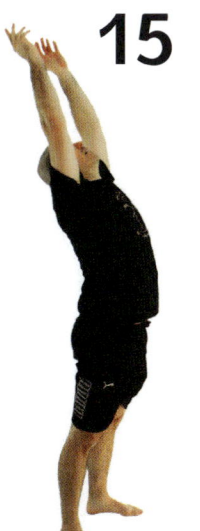
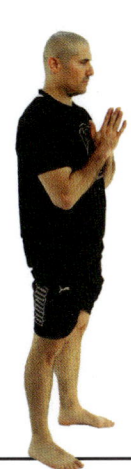

17 Inhale. Transition to side kneeling and exhale for relaxation while in position

18 Side kneeling - inhale. Transition to other side and exhale for relaxation while in position

19 Arms in front, transfer body weight to hands

20 Bend elbows outward and place knees on arms

21 Transfer body weight to the hands until feet break contact with ground

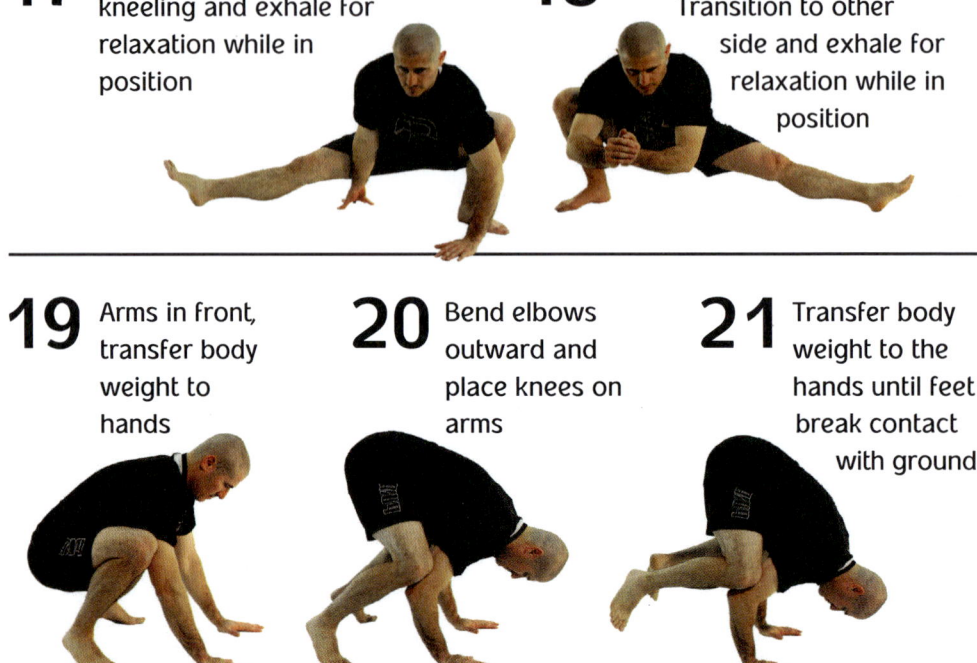

4.5 Practicing basic movement patterns

By practicing basic movement patterns we can identify and then remove limitations to our mobility. Each of the exercises should be treated as tools for evaluating and identifying exercisers' lack of ability and limitations. Overcoming limitations or difficulties improves exercisers' abilities, removes pain, and improves functioning and general feeling. On the other hand, the inability to perform a specific exercise may indicate a problem (a weak link in the mobility chain) and an existing - or imminent - functional problem.

Every exerciser may have factors that limit mobility. Possible causes of these factors are:

1. Poor posture
2. Flexibility issues - limitation in tissue length
3. Muscular issues - limitations in strength
4. Nervous issues - awareness, understanding movement
5. Pathological issues - limitations or pain

When one body limb or other part of the kinetic chain compensates for another limb, this indicates a limitation in mobility.

Functional approach - It is important to take into consideration factors that may limit mobility when performing exercises and to adapt each exercise to the individual body's structure, abilities and limitations. To conclude the warm-up, a stick is used for performing exercises.

The squat movement pattern
The aim of the exercise is to evaluate mobility of the ankle, knee and hip as well as to move and keep hands above the head and stabilize the lumbar and thoracic spine during the squat.

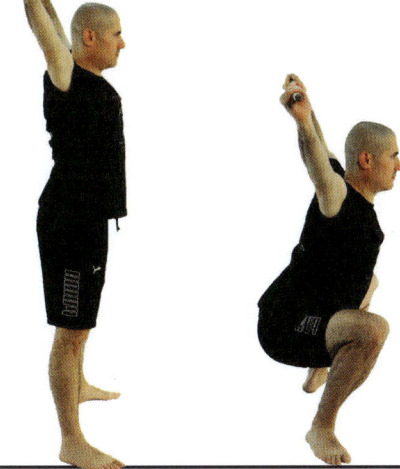

- No pain during the movement
- The spine moves toward the vertical
- The hips are below knee level
- Knees are in line with the feet
- Hold stick above the feet

Lifting movement pattern
The aim of the exercise is to evaluate posture, hip mobility and flexibility as well as the ability to maintain the spine in a natural, stable position.

- No pain during the movement
- Stick and body remain stable, no movement in the hip and spine
- The spine moves toward the horizontal

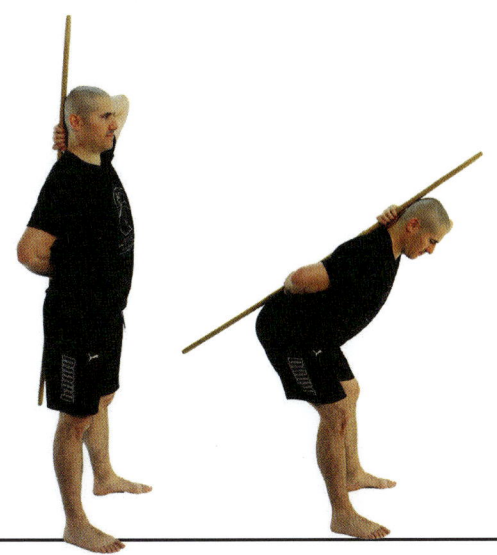

Lunge movement pattern

The aim of the exercise is to evaluate mobility and stability of the ankle and hip, knee stability, hip flexibility, and stability of the body in an asymmetrical position.

- No pain during the movement
- The spine moves toward the vertical, head above pelvis
- Stick and body remain stable
- Rear knee touches the floor

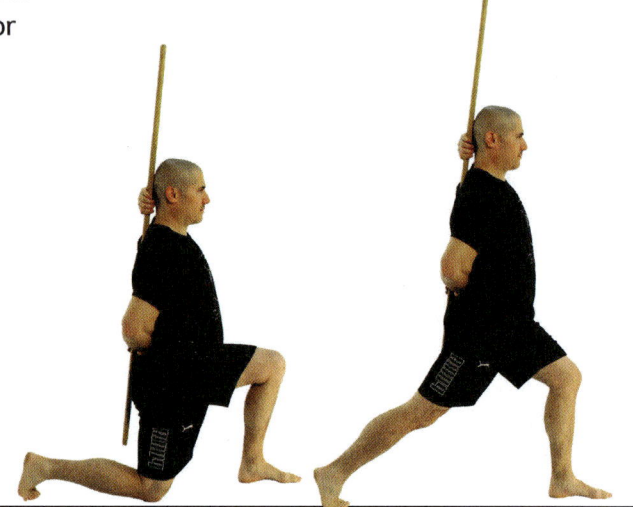

Spinal stability

The aim of the exercise is to evaluate spinal stability while opposing limbs move.

- No pain during the movement
- Stick and body remain stable

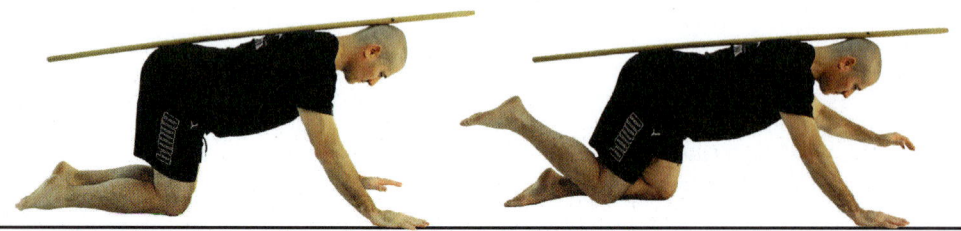

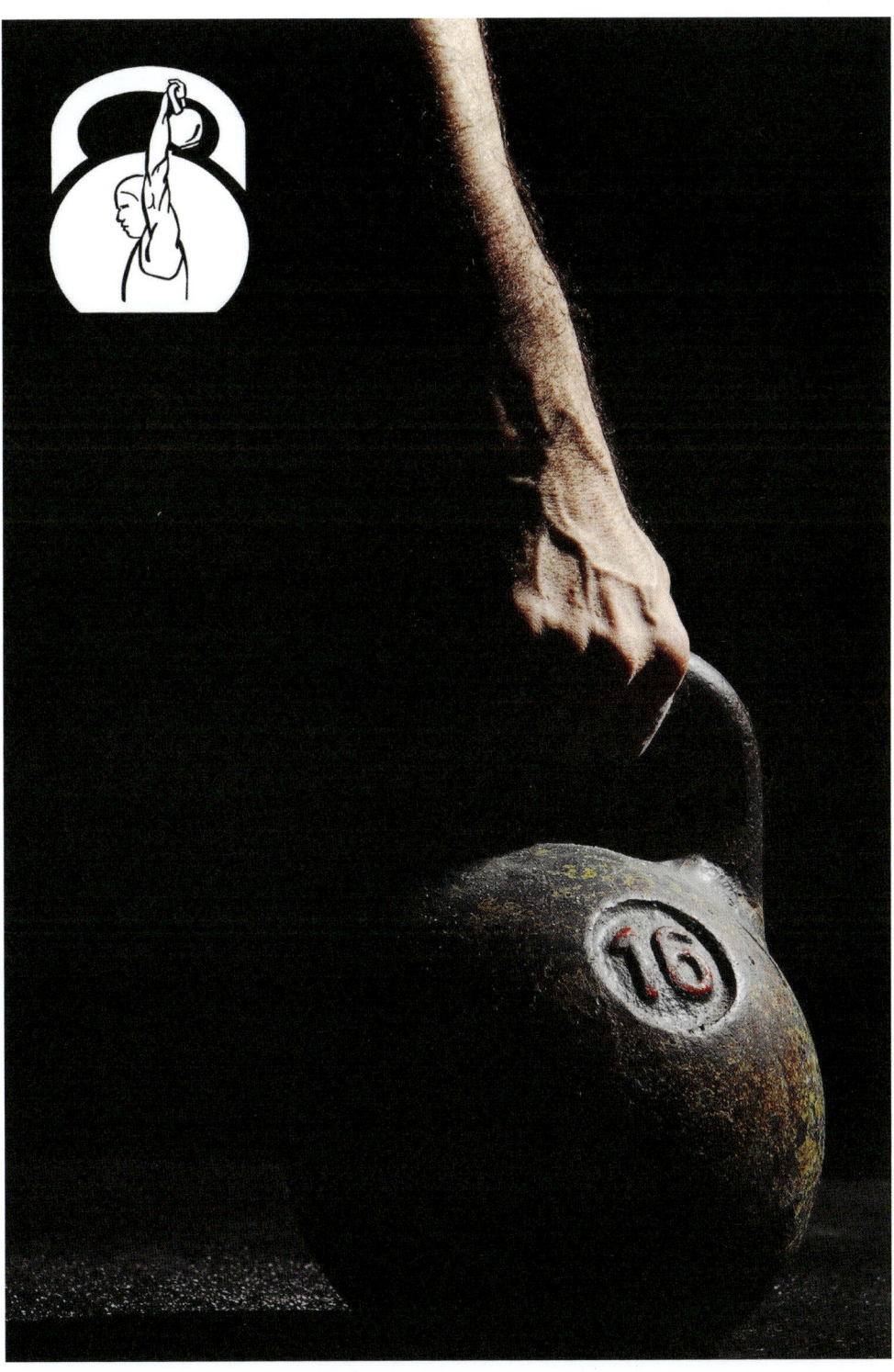

Get up

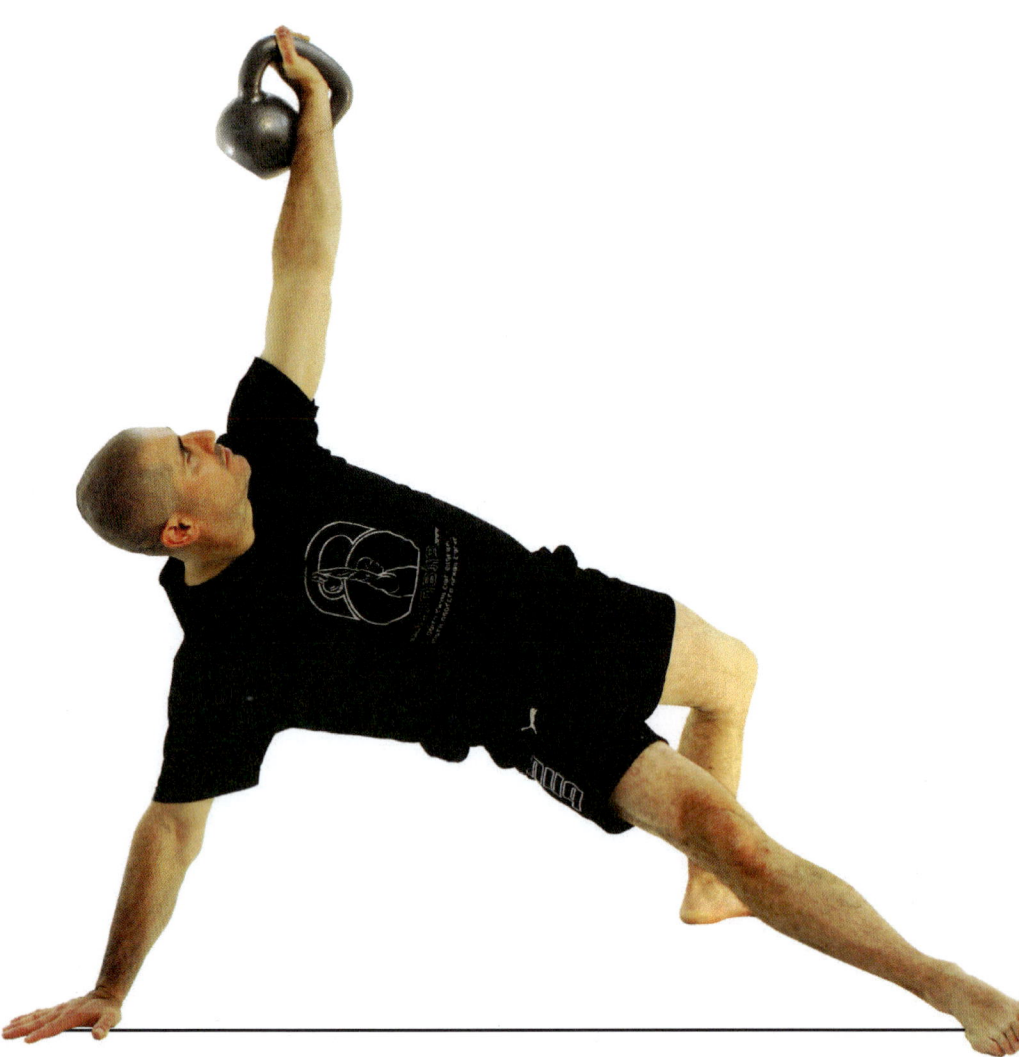

000 0000 | 48

4.6 Kettlebell exercises

4.6.1 Get up

Get up is actually our test of the entire body's stabilizing and mobility abilities, strength (to move, stabilize or delay), flexibility, equilibrium (or lack of equilibrium), coordination and kinesthesis (sensations of body part location and body state) during movement.

The exercise is composed of six stages. It is possible to stop at each stage and focus on it individually, in order to improve a weak component of movement or stabilization, and then to reconnect the stages into one kinetic sequence.

The joints involved in the exercise: foot, ankle, knee, hip, pelvis, spine, scapula, shoulder, elbow, wrist.

* During the exercise some of the joints are required to change roles from immobility (stability) to mobility and vice versa.

The safe way to begin the exercise:

1 Face the kettlebell, hold it with the closer hand and place the other hand on top of it.

2 Shift onto your back.

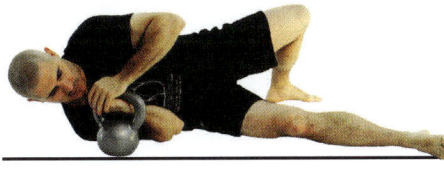

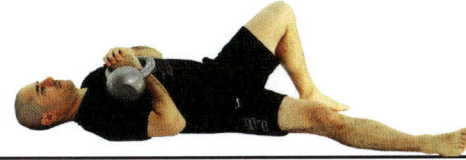

3 Push the kettlebell upward.

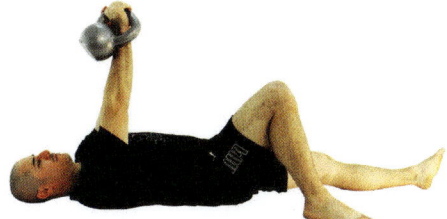

Lunge Get-up

1

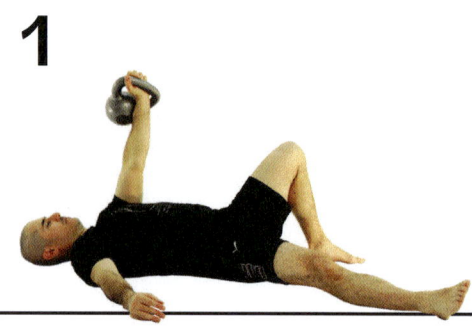

Starting position:
Left hand holds the kettlebell up, the free hand is 45 degrees from the hip. The left leg is bent and near the buttocks, the right leg is straight and faces slightly outward.

2 While exhaling, move from supine to sitting, roll sideways onto the right elbow.

3 While exhaling, push upward with the right arm until it is straight.

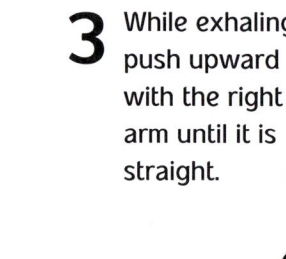

4 While inhaling, raise the pelvis.

5 While exhaling, move right leg behind, parallel to the right arm.

6 While inhaling, move to a one-leg kneeling position.

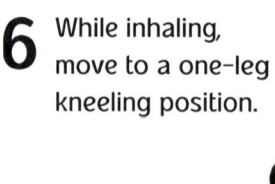

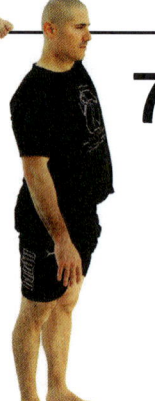

7 While exhaling, move from kneeling to standing; right leg moves to the left leg.

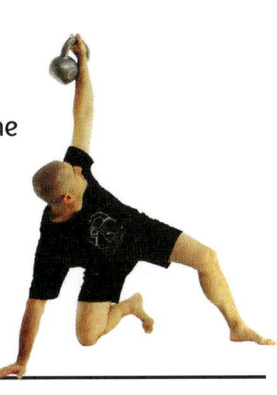

8 While inhaling, right leg moves to the rear and kneels.

9 While exhaling, the right hand returns to the floor.

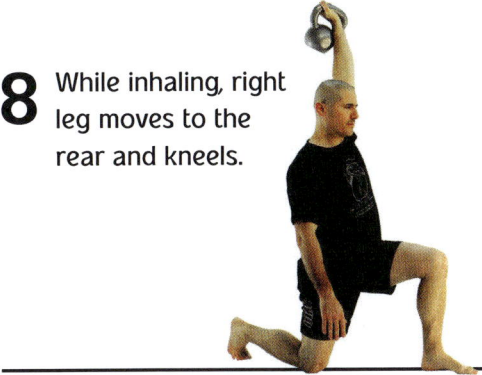

10 While exhaling, the right leg straightens forward.

11 While exhaling, the pelvis lowers to the floor.

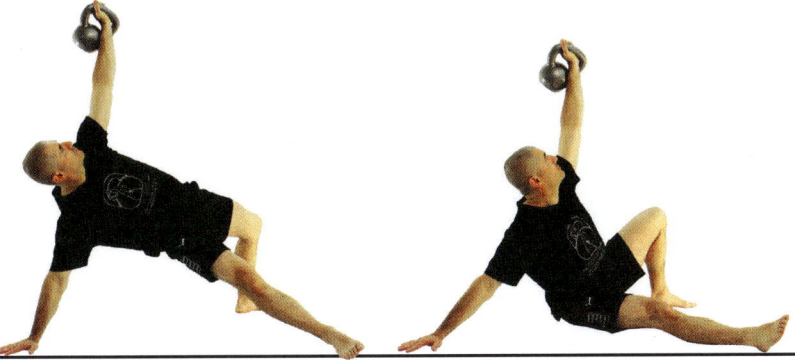

12 While exhaling, rest on right elbow.

13 While exhaling, carefully roll back to a supine position.

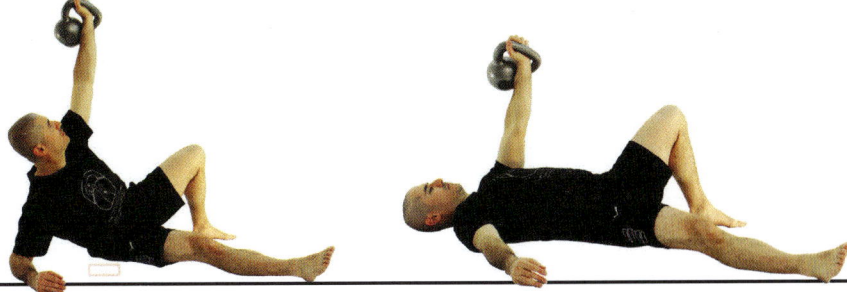

Exercises for variation:
Squat Get-up

1

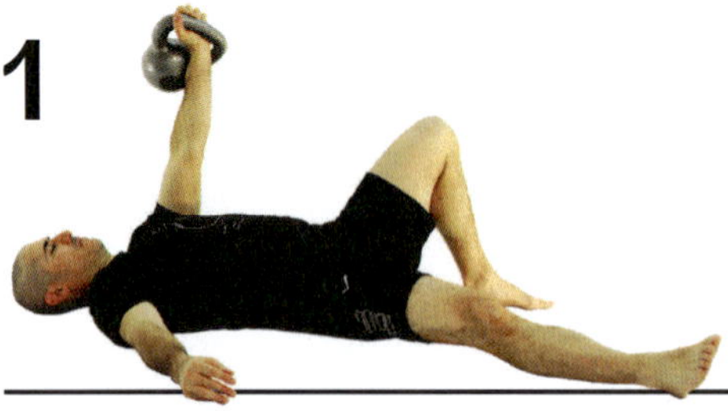

2

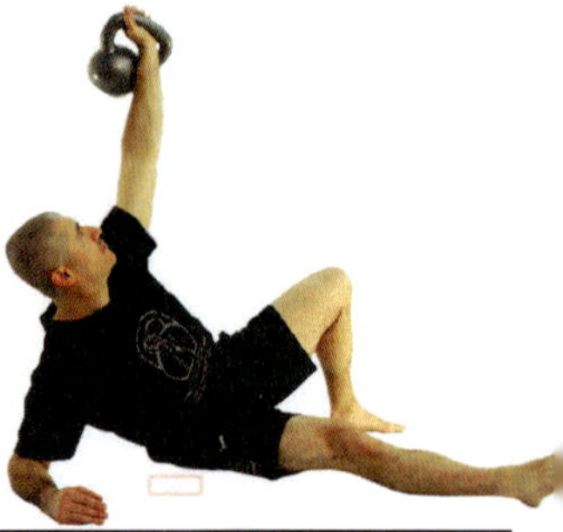

3

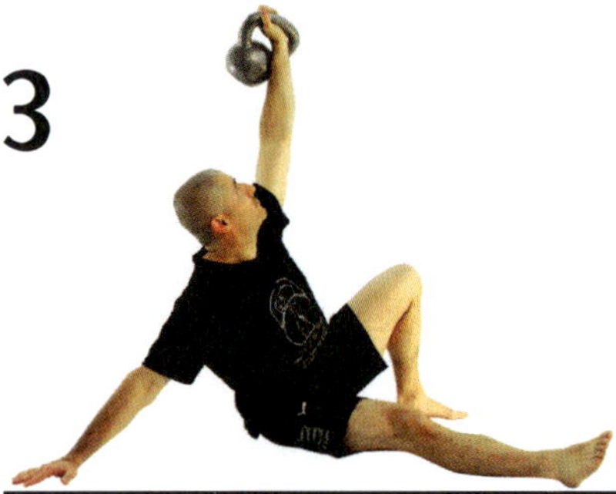

4

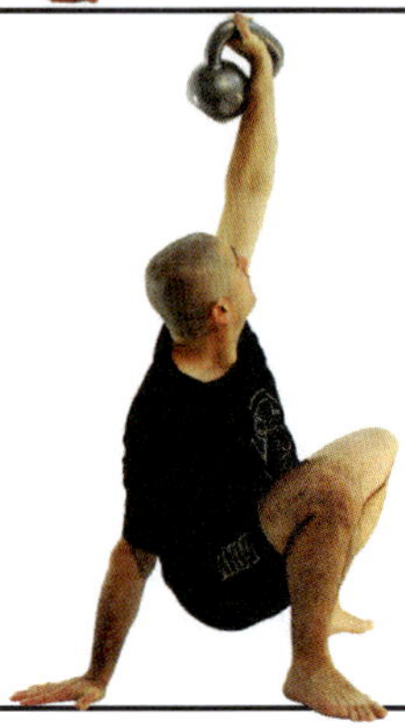

5

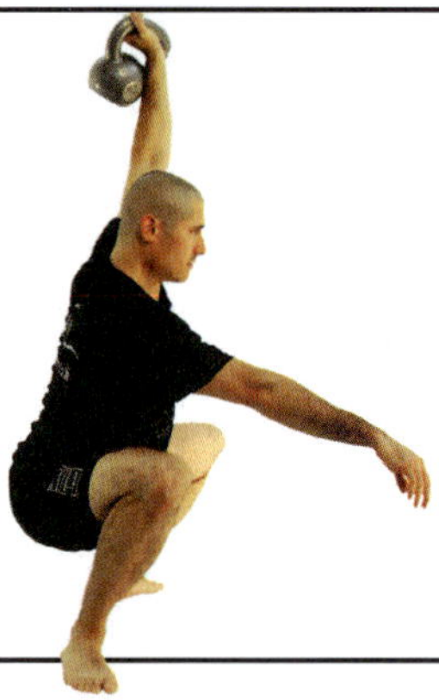

6

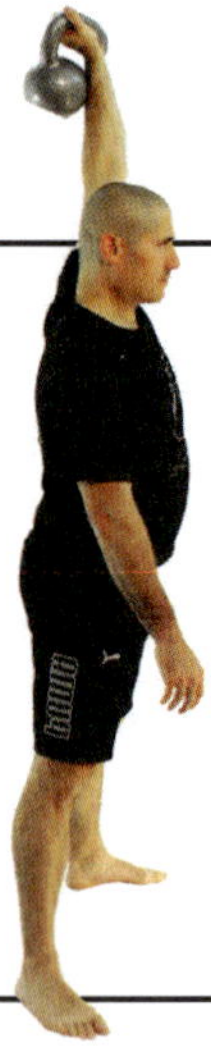

2H Get up (getting up without using hands)

1

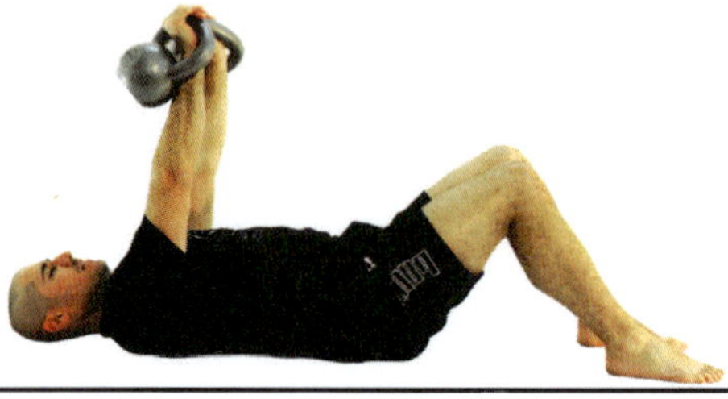

2

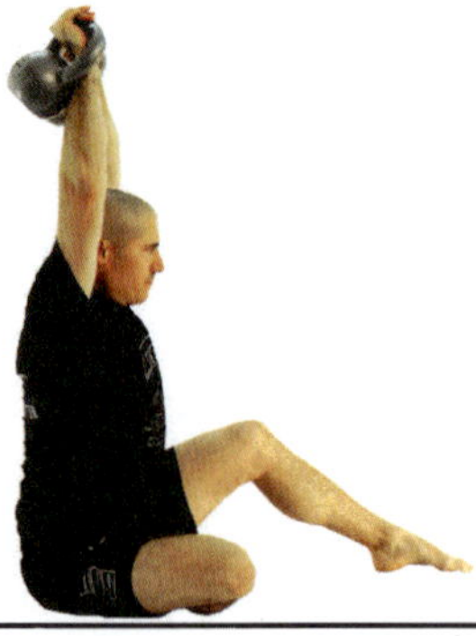

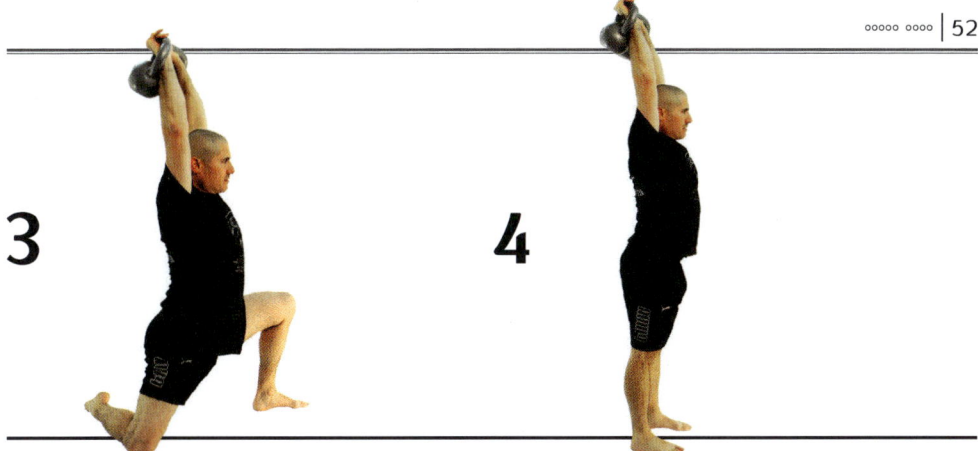

3

4

Plank Get up (getting up through the side)

1

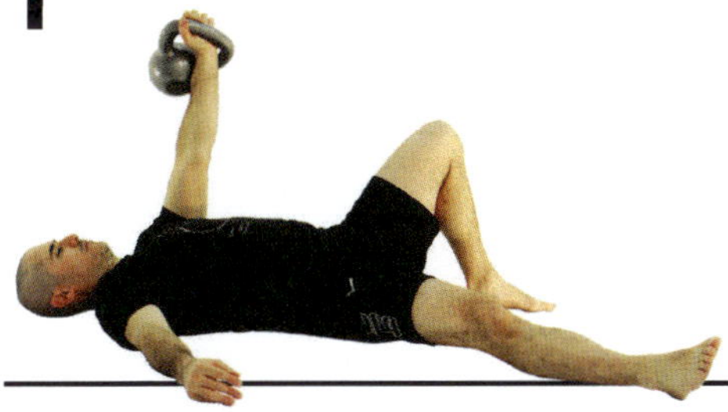

2

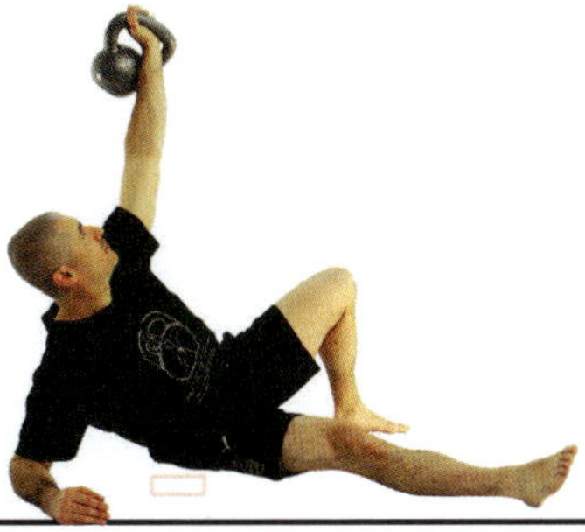

3

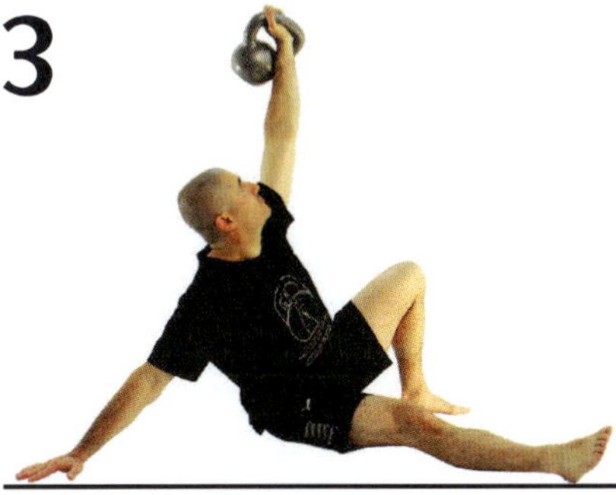

4

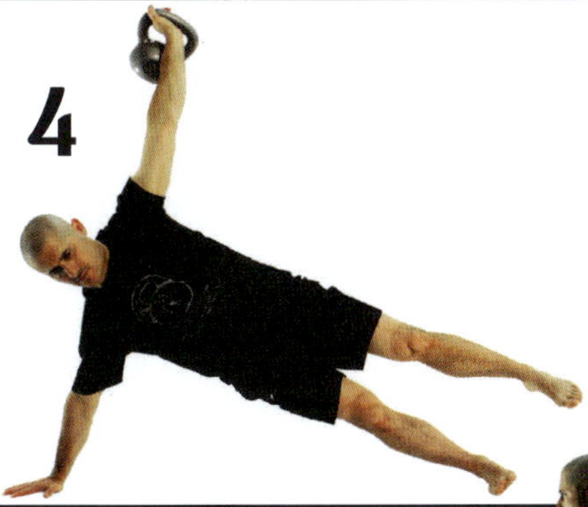

5

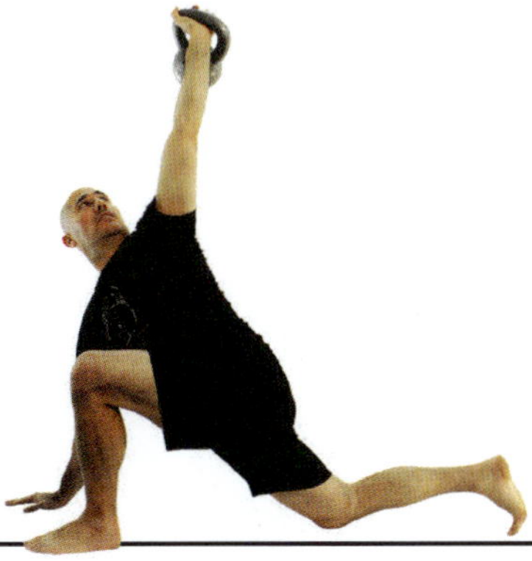

6

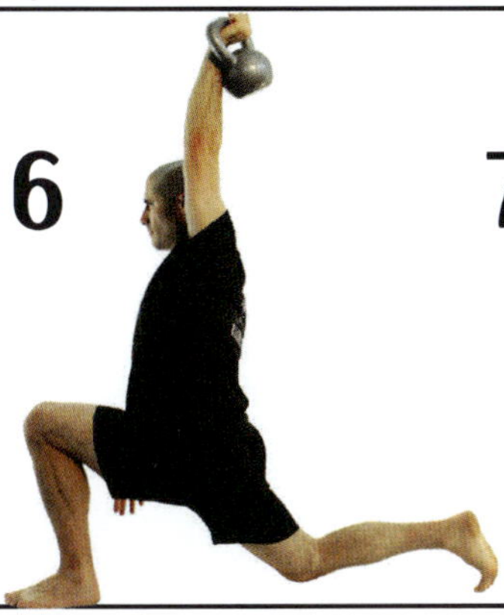

7

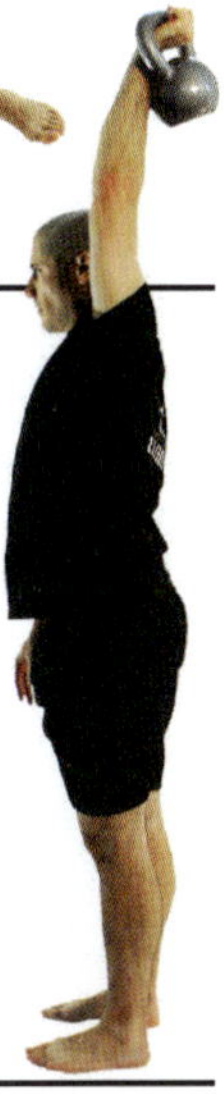

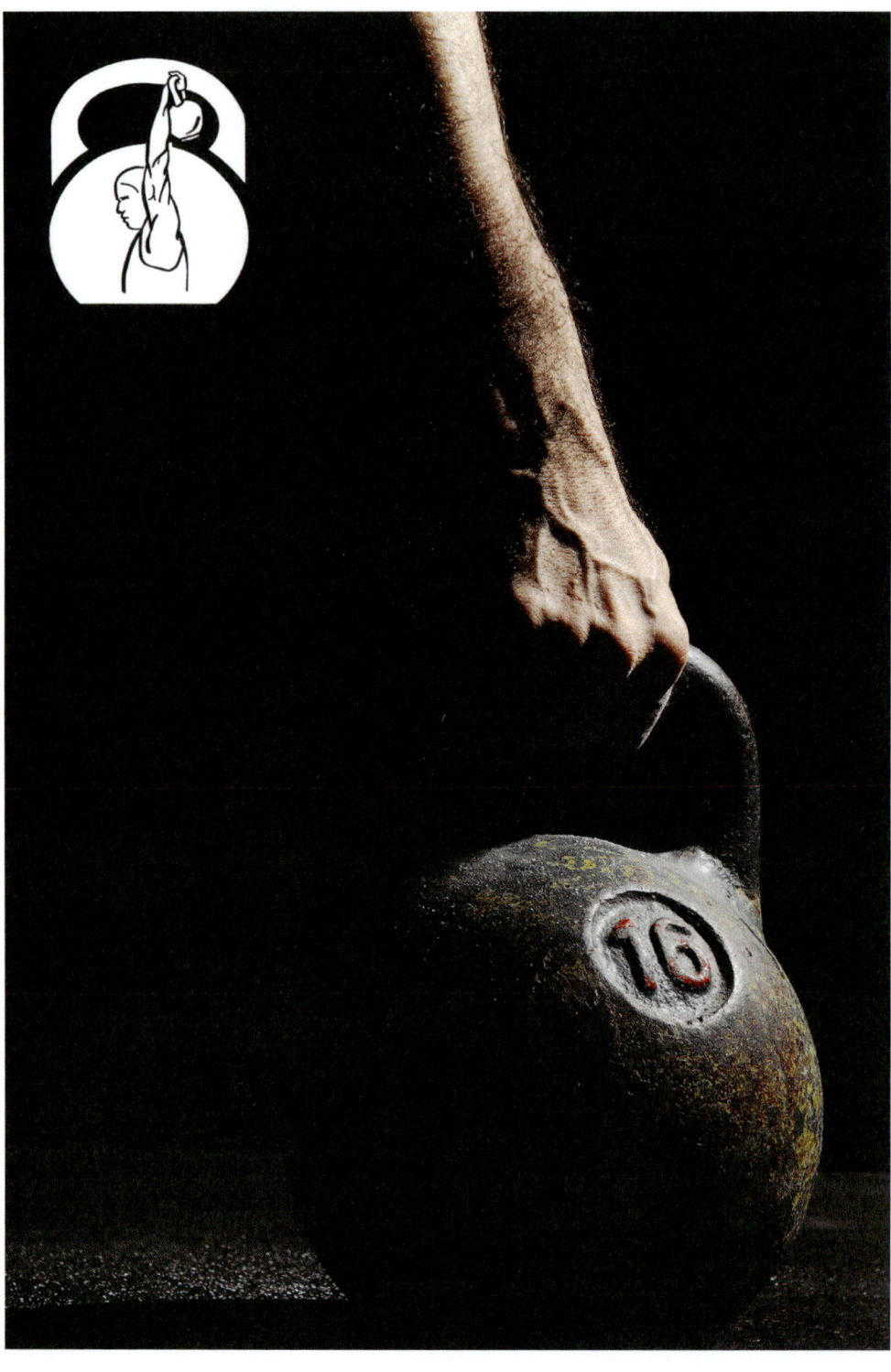

Dead-lift

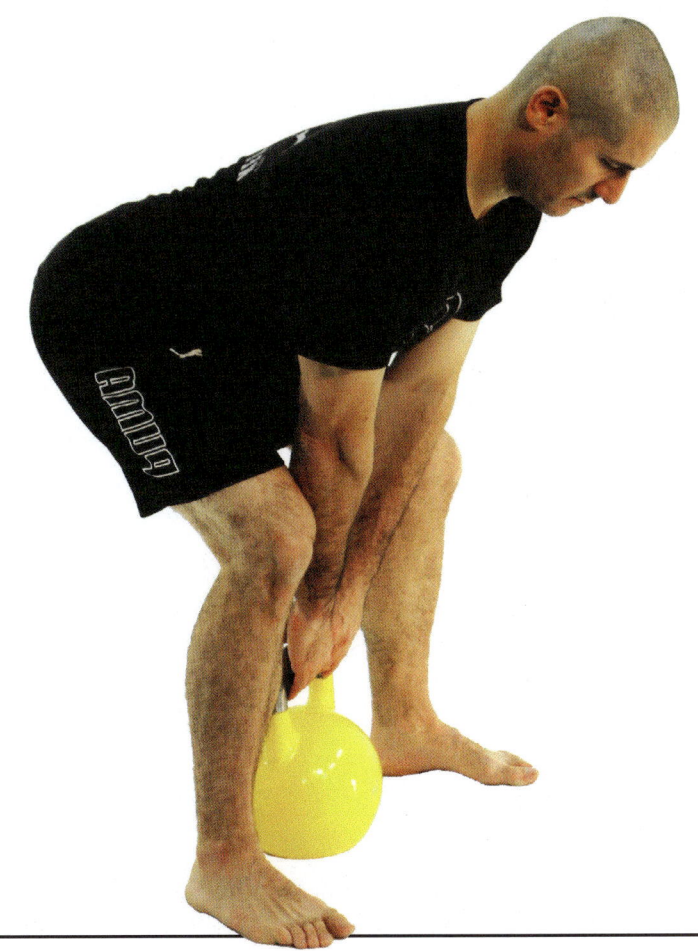

4.6.2 Dead-lift

The dead-lift is the key exercise. It is an exercise based on a natural body movement pattern and is necessary for maintaining our health and our functionality. It teaches us how to move our body efficiently during swinging exercises, and is a preparatory exercise for all other swinging exercises (snatch, clean, swing).

Mobility - joints that are supposed to move: ankle, knee, hip.

Stabilization - joints that are not supposed to move: foot, pelvis, spine, scapula/shoulder, elbow, wrist.

Three important things in the dead-lift exercise:

1. Elongation to the rear (hip mobility).
2. Spine remains in a natural position (spinal stability).
3. The kettlebell is located on the body's center line of gravity.

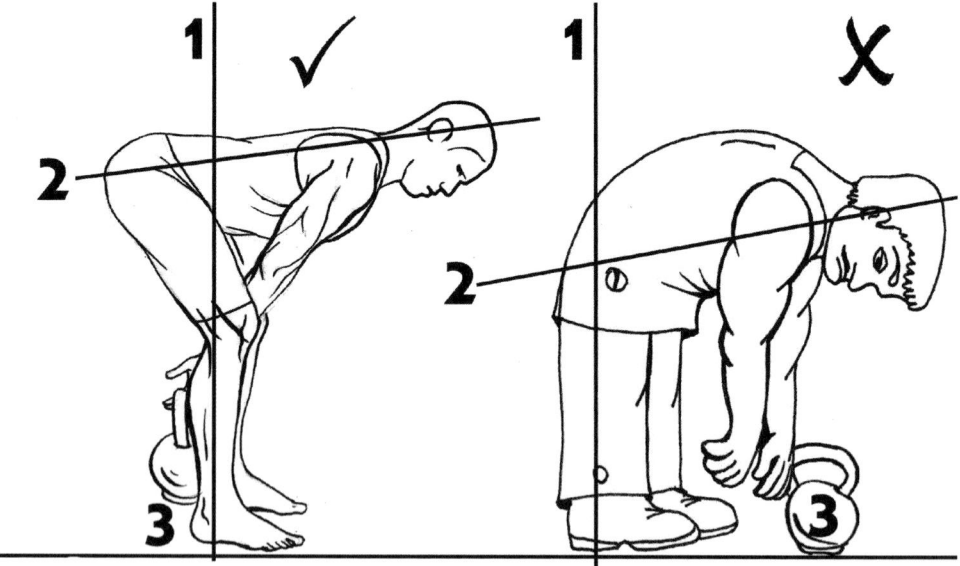

Dead-lift

1 While exhaling, keep the back stable and return to a standing position.

2 While inhaling, the sitting bones (pubis) lengthen to the rear, with a slight flexion of the knees.

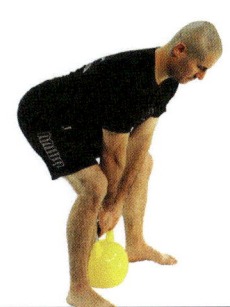

Common errors and adaptations:

1. Do not flex the spine - keep it in a natural position.
2. Make sure the kettlebell is not too far from the center line of gravity or from the base of support - place the kettlebell in line with the heels.
3. Lack of flexibility in the hips may cause the pelvis to tilt to the rear, which will cause flexion of the lumbar spine (which is supposed to remain stable). Until we develop the desired range of movement in the hips, we can take a step to bring the kettlebell closer to us.

1   **2**   **3**

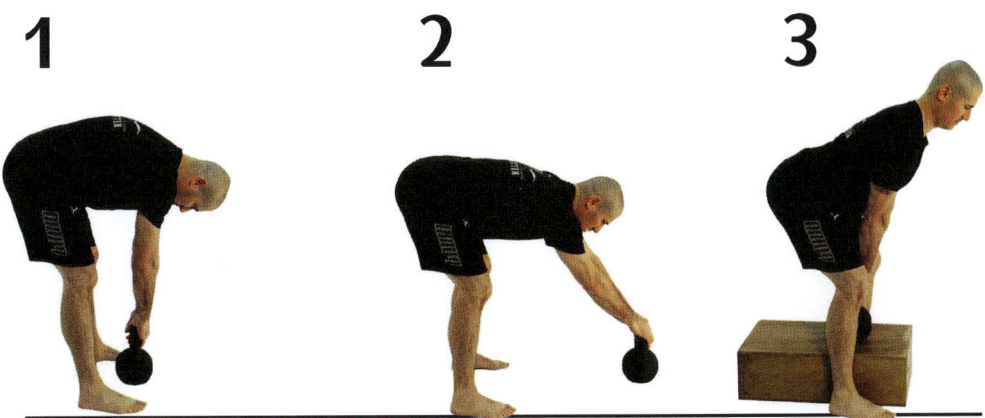

Exercise variations:

Good morning

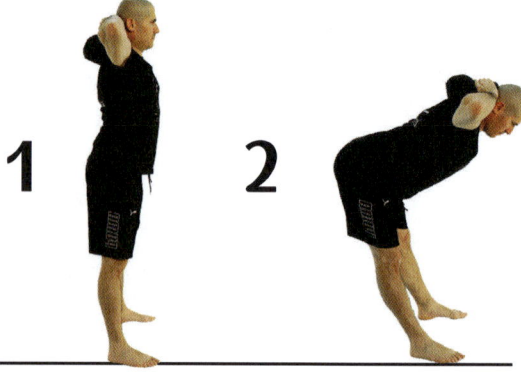

1   2

Single leg dead-lift

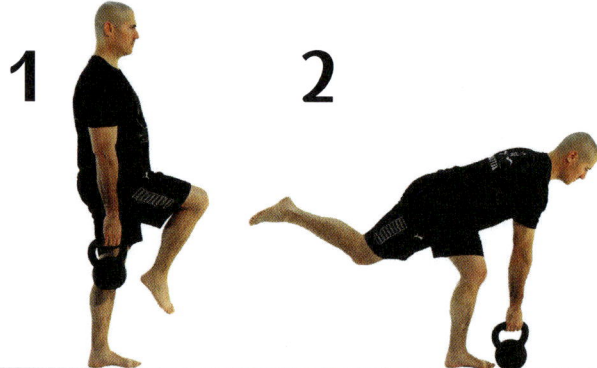

1   2

Single leg
dead-lift
+ pull

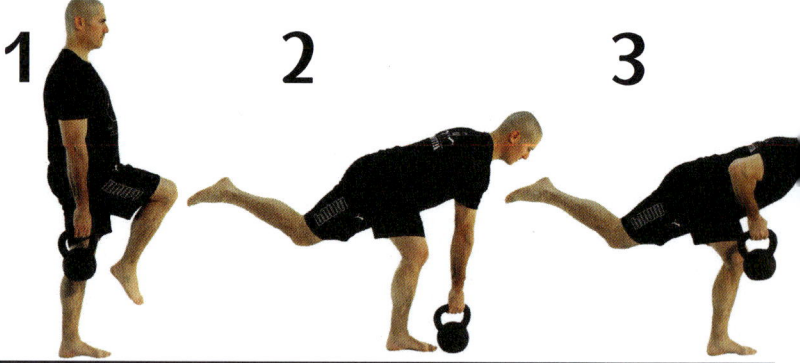

1   2   3

Suitcase dead-lift

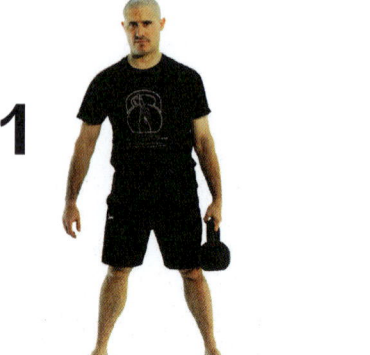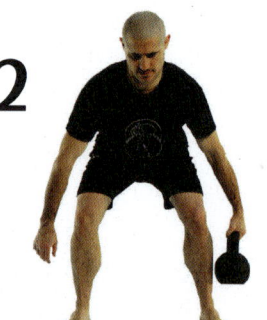

1   2

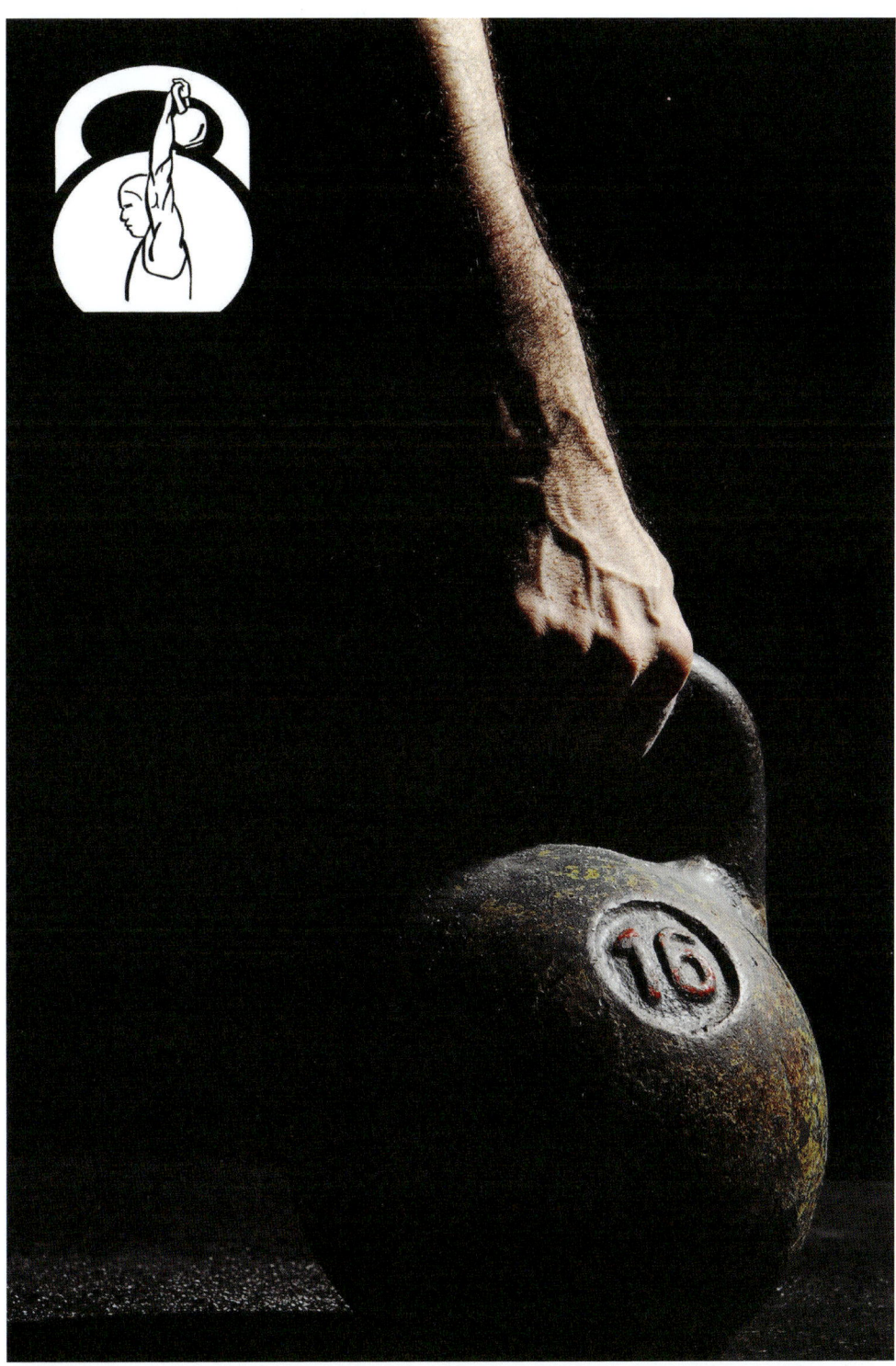

Preparation for snatch, clean and swing

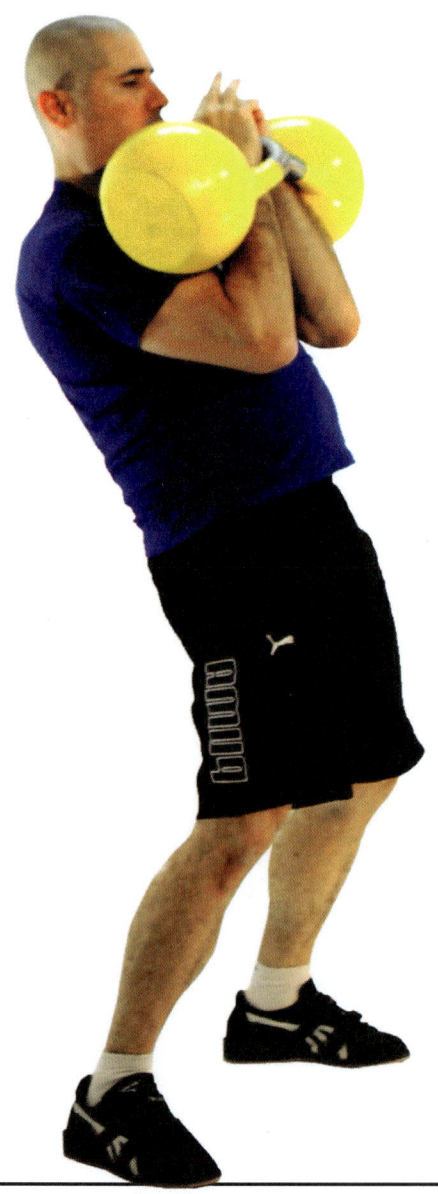

4.6.3 Preparation for snatch, clean and swing

Safe lifting

In contrast to the way we lift kettlebells in the dead-lift exercise, where they are placed between our legs, in the snatch, clean and swing exercises the kettlebells are located far from the sitting bones (pubis bone). Arms are straight on the kettlebell handle and like cocking a spring, we send the sitting bones far from the handle, so that a light pull of the arms will make the kettlebell move between the legs and from there it can be swung up.

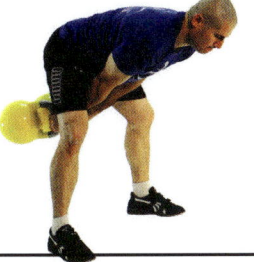 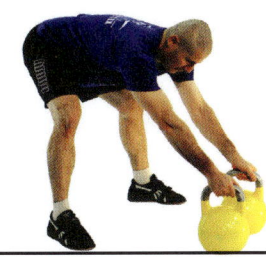

Rack position (intermediate stance)

The rack position is the intermediate stance of the long cycle between the clean and the jerk, and the starting position for the squat and press exercises.

Gripping the kettlebell in the rack position: the handle is placed diagonally on the wrist, thumb pointing to the rear, fingers (closed/open) behind the handle, elbow touching the ribs/pelvis, and pelvis tilted forward with legs straight.

Rack position – Weight lifting vs. kettlebells

In weight lifting, the bar is placed on the palm of the hand, which is lying on the clavicle, and the elbows are lifted. Kettlebells, in contrast, are placed on the wrist which rests on the elbow, the pelvis or the ribs. Each location varies exercise performance and emphases.

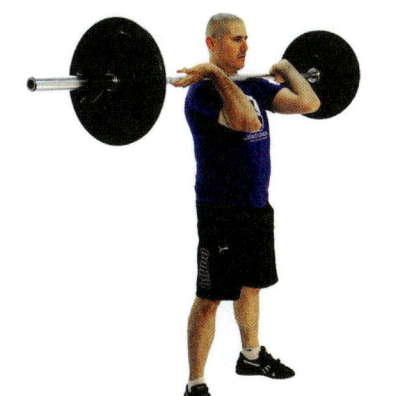 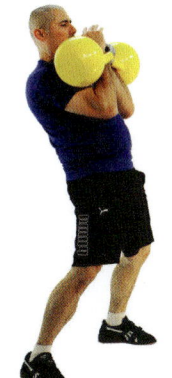

Hook grip

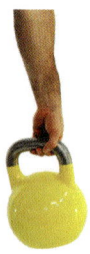

The hook grip is used with snatch, clean and swing exercises.
Gripping the kettlebell handle on the downswing: the handle is placed
on the outermost joint of the fingers, with the thumb locking it in place
from above.

Lock-out position (straight arm stance)

The lock-out position is created by straightening the arm upward at the end of the
press, push, clean and jerk, and snatch exercises.
The kettlebell handle during and at the conclusion of the snatch: Shift the handle
diagonally onto the wrist, with the thumb pointing to the rear and fingers behind
the handle.

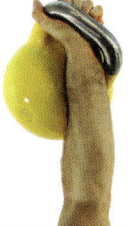 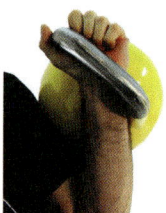 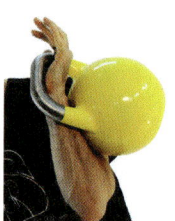

Horn position 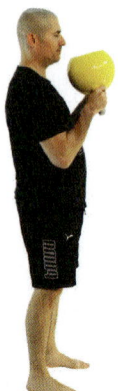   Bottom-up position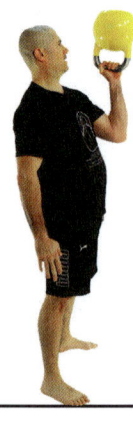

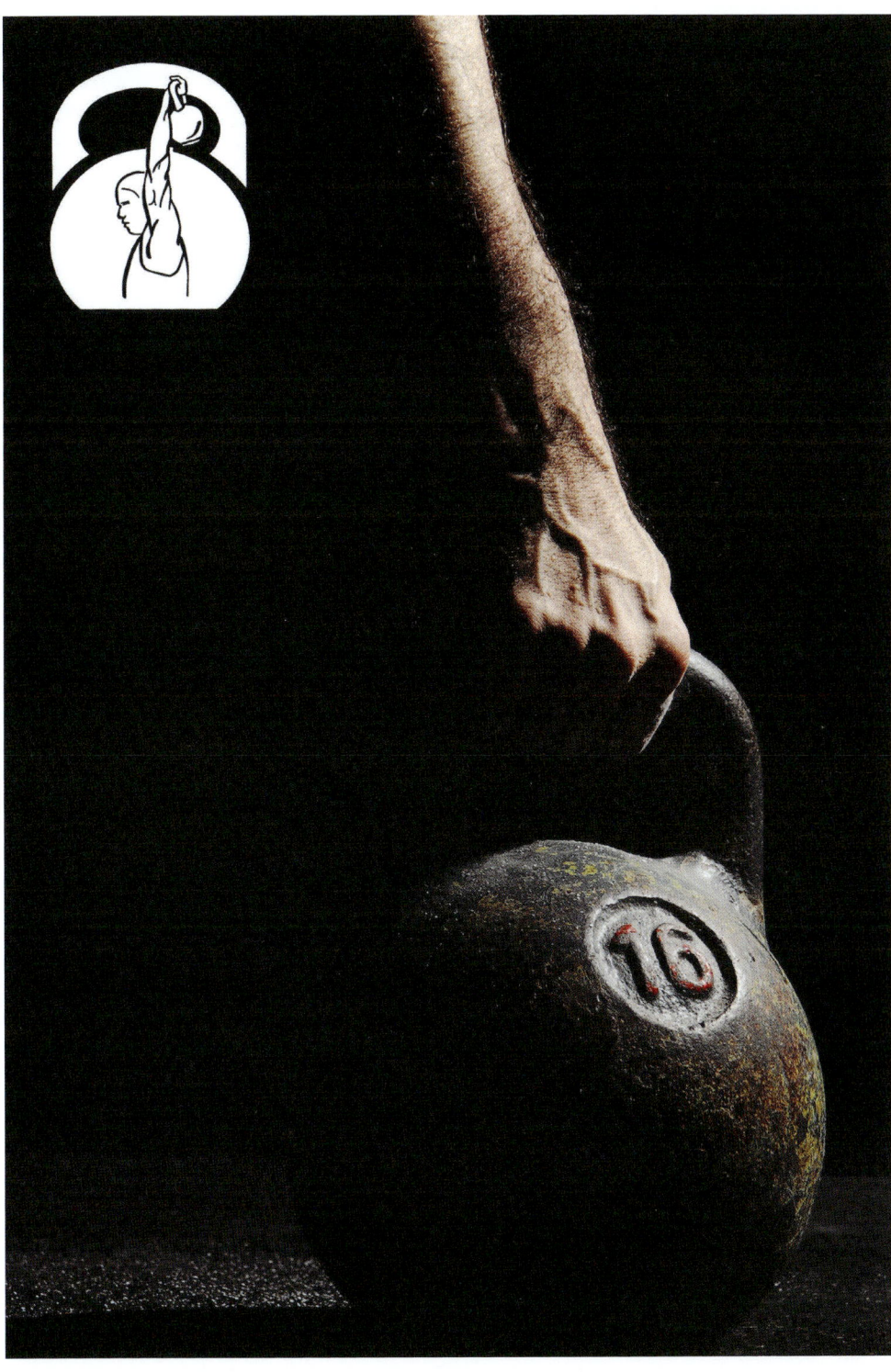

Swing

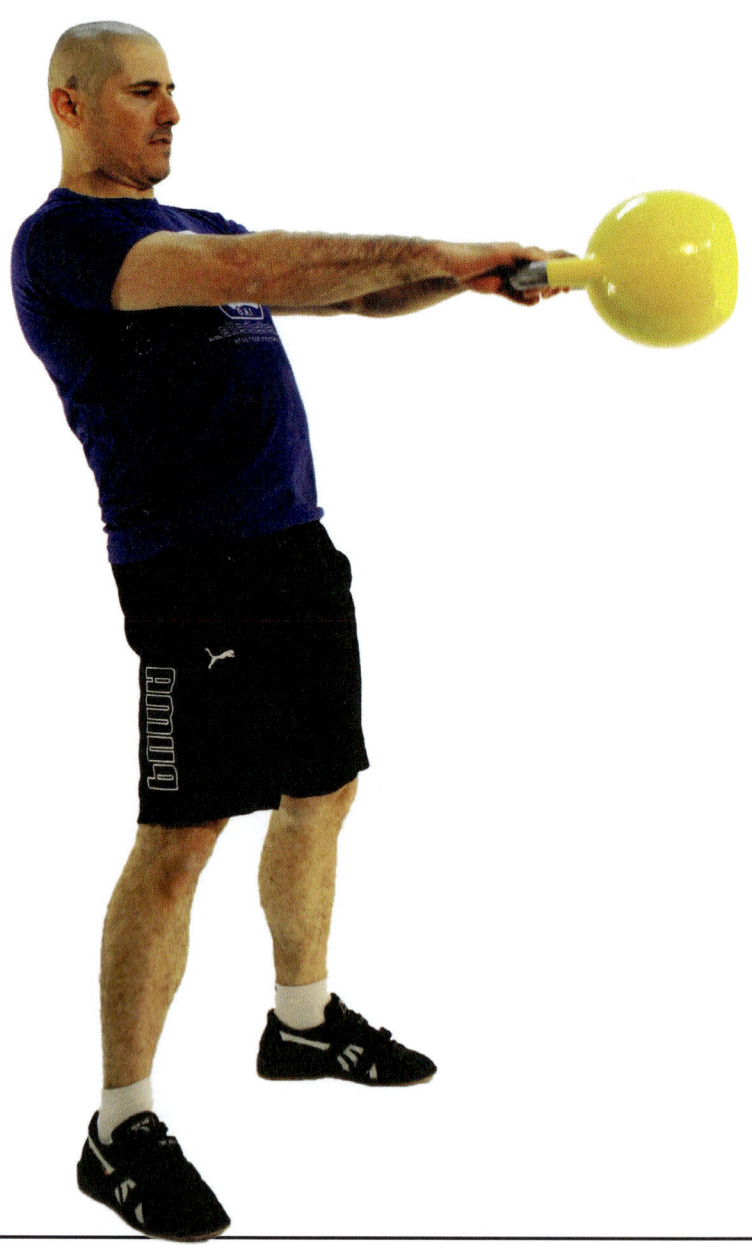

4.6.4 Swing

The swing is a dynamic movement exercise and the first of other swing exercises. It is a basic exercise for other snatch and clean exercises.

2H swing (with both hands)

1 Push the sitting bones backward, while slighting flexing the knees, and let the kettlebell fall between the feet. Stabilize the pelvis and spine.

2 Push the feet against the floor and the pelvis forward and upward to an erect standing position. With pelvic momentum, the arms become "weightless" and swing upward.

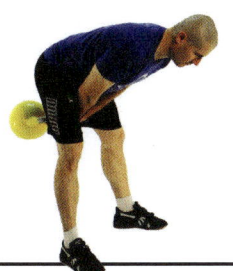

Common errors and adaptations:

Do not bend the knees forward (this is not a squatting pattern) - lengthen to the rear through the buttocks.

Do not bend the spine - maintain the spine in its normal position.

Do not use the shoulder girdle for swinging - the arms must be relaxed. Pelvic momentum makes the arms "weightless" and they fly upward.

1   **2**   **3**

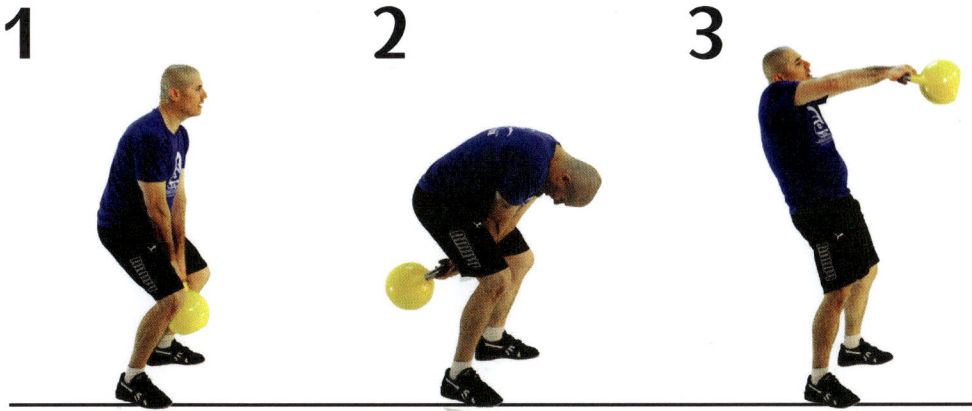

Varying the exercise:

1H swing (with one arm)

H2H swing (swing from hand to hand)

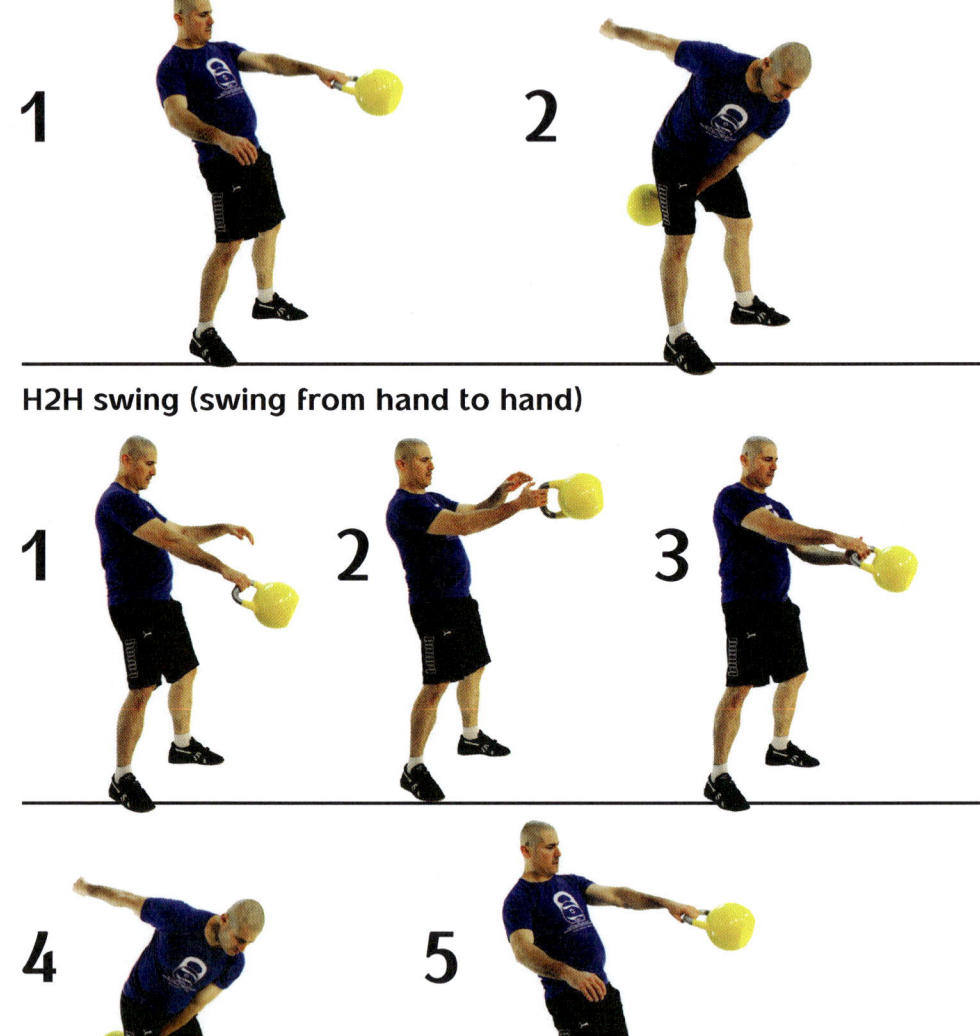

Switching hands in the H2H swing is done at the high point, at the zero point between concluding the kettlebell swing and allowing gravity to pull the kettlebell back down again.

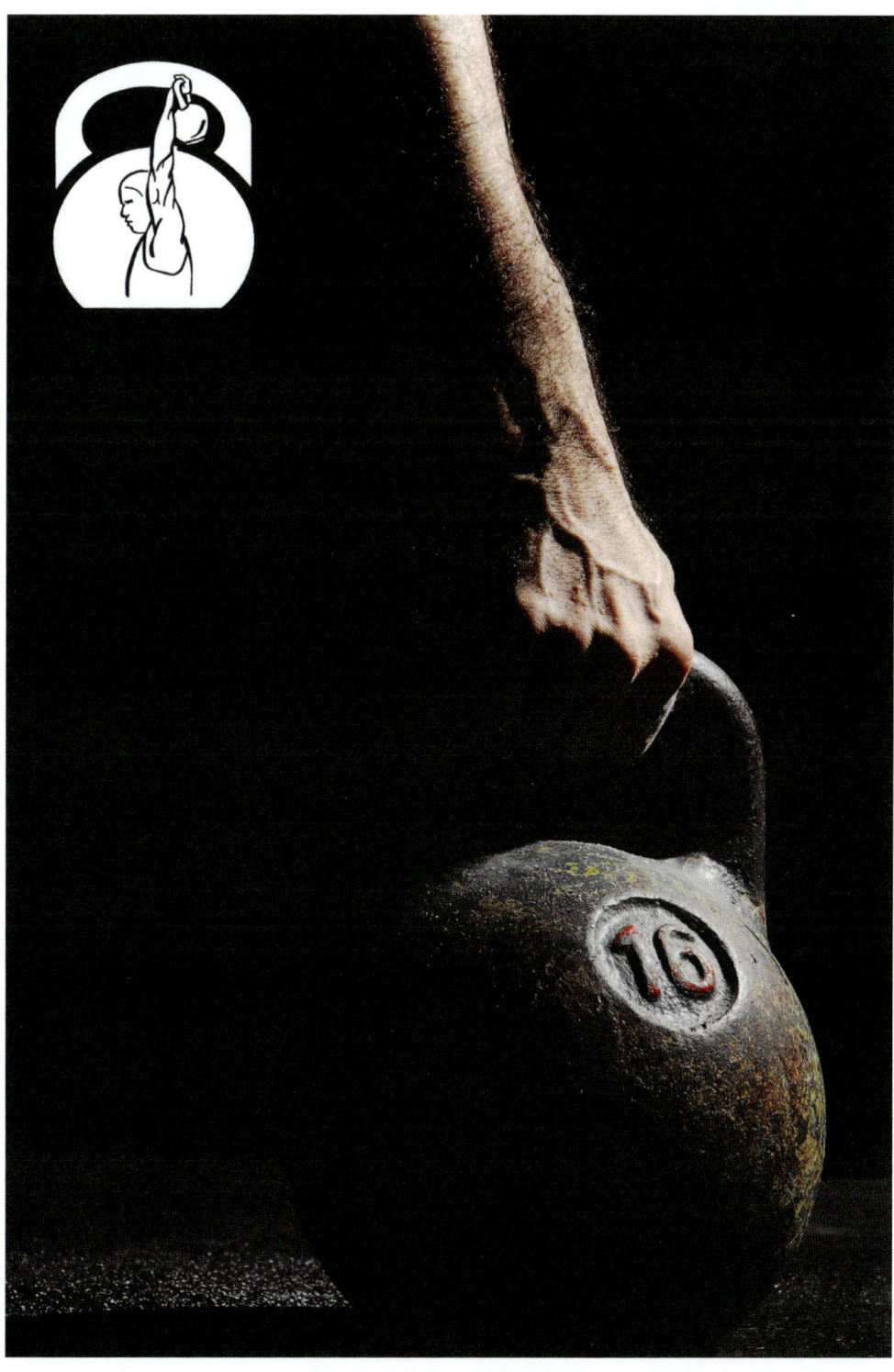

Clean

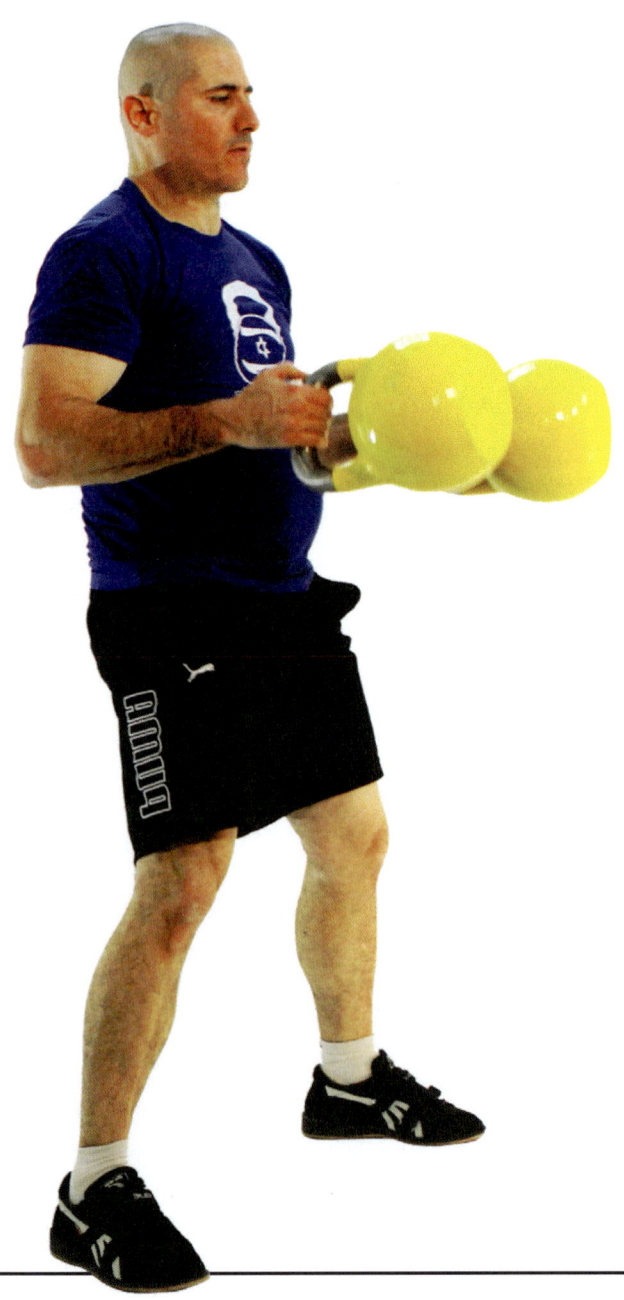

4.6.5 Clean

Clean is a swinging exercise intended to bring the kettlebell from the floor to the rack position easily, efficiently, safely and cleanly.

Clean

Bringing the kettlebell to the starting point using a safe swing (see page 59)

Starting position

Rack position

1 Lower the kettlebell –
Tilt the body back and let the kettlebell fall between the legs

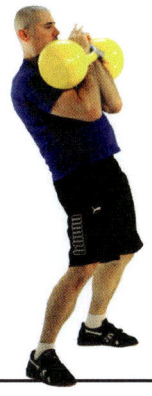
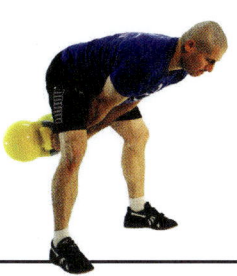

2 Swing - during the swing (lifting the hip and heel on the swinging arm side) the arm should maintain contact with the ribs/hip

3 While swinging, rotate the traversing wrist so that the kettlebell moves around the wrist, and pull the elbow toward the hip.

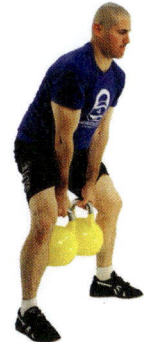
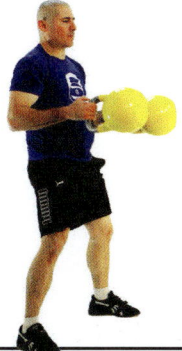
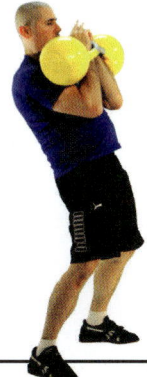

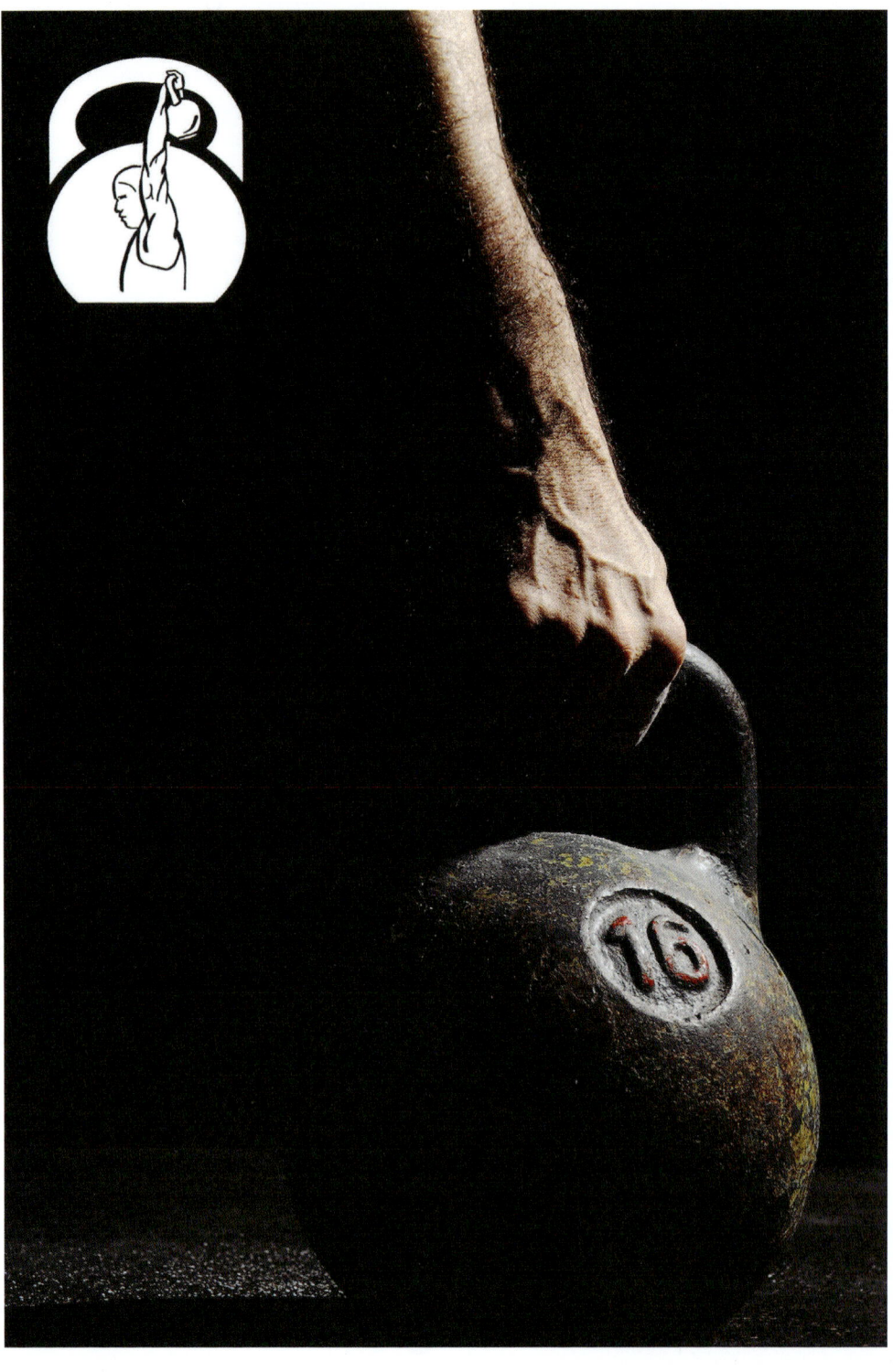

Squat

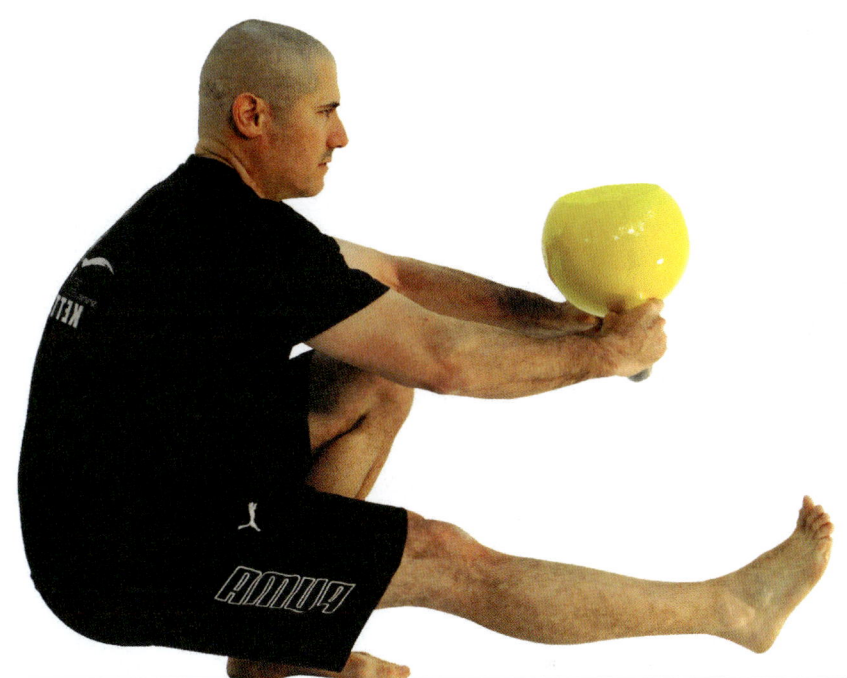

4.6.6 Squat

The squat is not the classic movement pattern of the kettlebell world (swinging exercises are based on the dead-lift). But the squat is a basic supplementary exercise that helps to build general body strength and improve athletic ability, which will then be reflected in other exercises. The exercise is essential for maintaining our functionality, mobility and stability and thus our health. If we compare our body to an automobile, then the dead-lift is our chassis (how we move our bodies), and the squat is the motor (the power to move our bodies).

Unlike dead-lift and swinging, the squat does not require extensive learning but to perform it optimally, it is important to identify and remove any factors that limit mobility.

Mobility - the joints that are supposed to move: Ankle, knee, hip

Stability - the joints that are not supposed to move: Foot, pelvis, spine, scapula, shoulder, elbow, wrist.

Squat

1 While inhaling/ holding the breath, push sitting bones back towards the heels. Keep the spine stable.

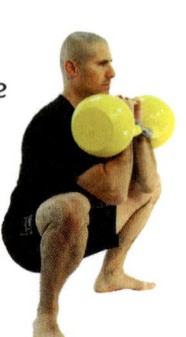

2 While exhaling, push feet against the floor and lead the buttocks forward and up, to an erect standing position.

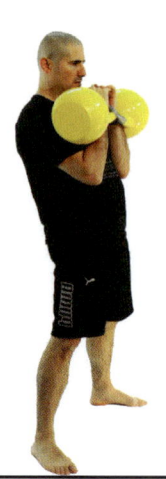

Common errors and adaptations

1. Do not let the knees collapse inward - keep the knees in line with the feet.
2. Do not flex the spine - keep the center strong.
3. To not let the buttocks rise - push from the feet.

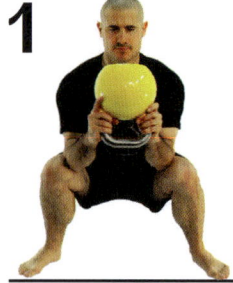 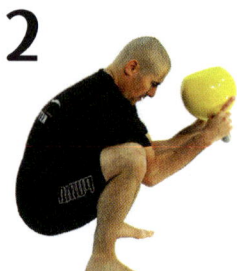 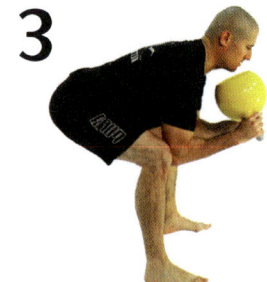

Exercise Variations

Squat goblet

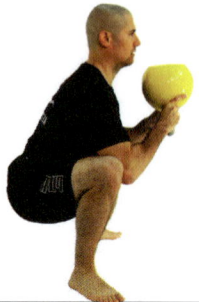 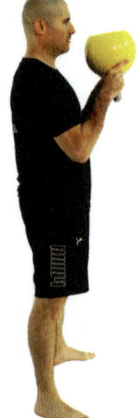

Jump squat

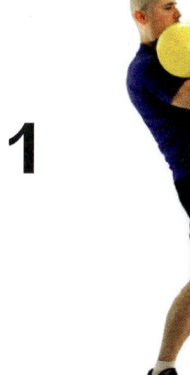

1

2

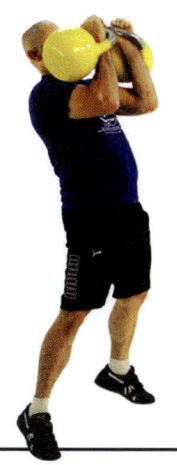

Overhead squat

1

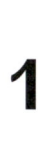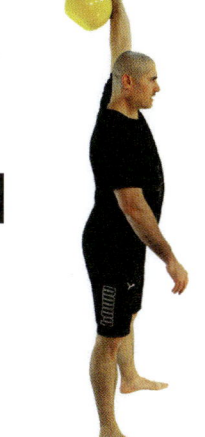

2

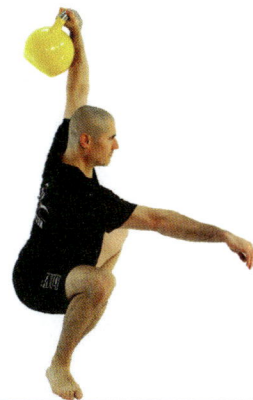

Pistol
(squat on one leg)

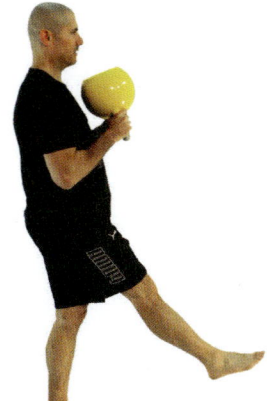

1

2

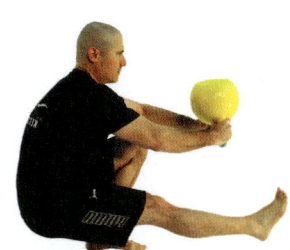

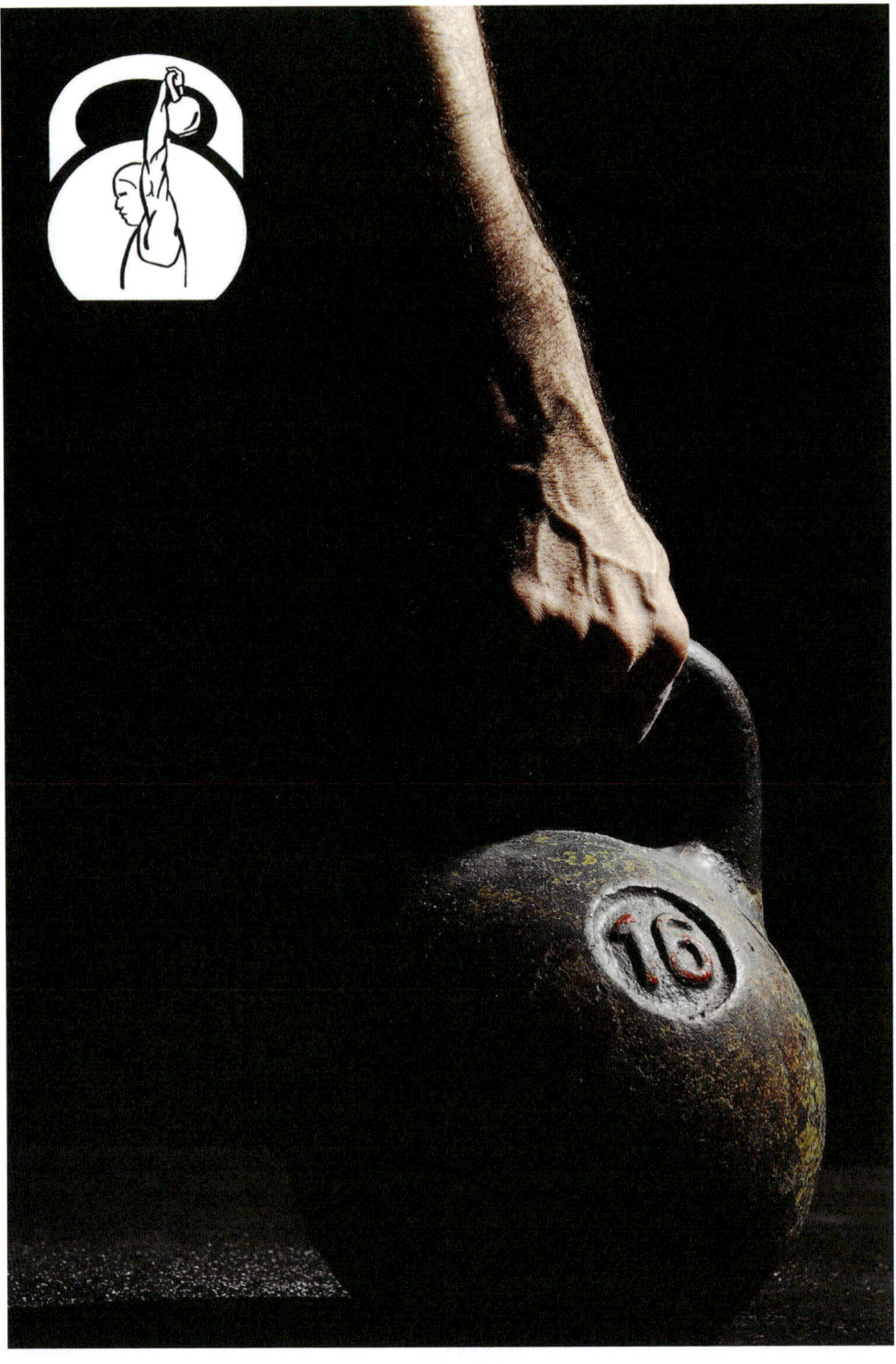

Press

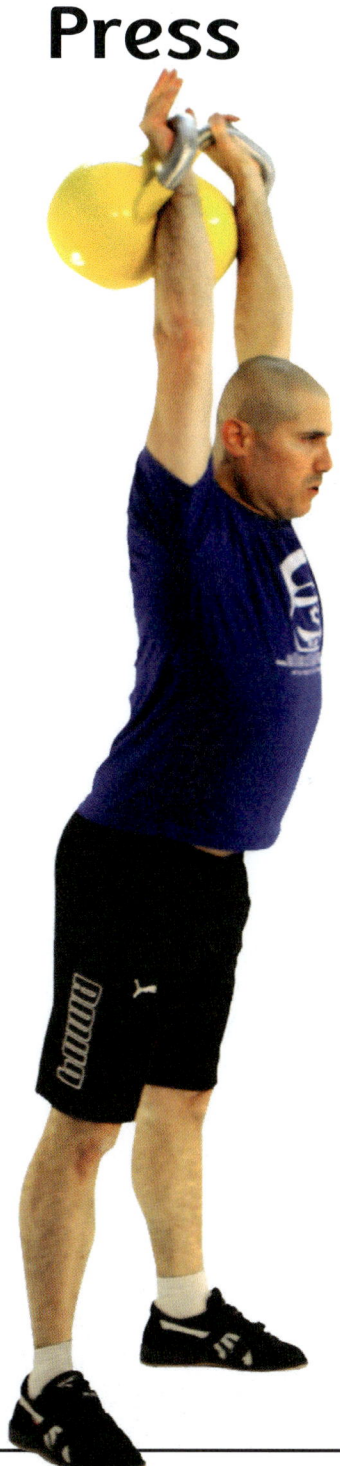

4.6.7 Press

The press is the basic pushing exercise in which we press the kettlebell from the rack position to above the head, with legs straight and arms straight up (lock-out position). It is also a preparatory exercise for push-press and jerk exercises.
Mobility - the joints that are supposed to move: scapula, shoulder, elbow.
Stabilization - the joints that are not supposed to move: foot, ankle, knee, hip, pelvis, spine, wrist.

Press

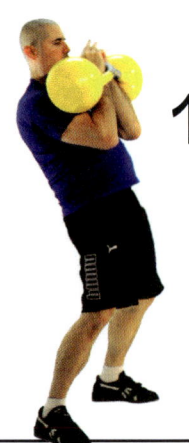

1 Press the kettlebell from the rack position to the lock-out position overhead.

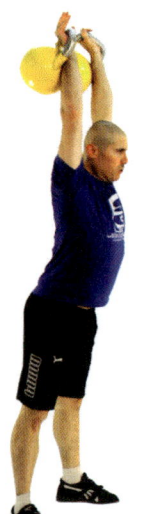

2 End with legs straight and arms straight up

As we progress from the press through the push-press to the jerk, we move from basic movement ability, which improves strength in the upper part of the body, to complex athletic ability and mobility exercise for the entire body (the mobilization power that comes from the legs and center of the body. Shoulder girdle strength is not significant and serves mainly to stabilize the kettlebell above the head). The exercise requires explosive power (strength + speed) and coordination (agility + reaction time). Pushing ability in the jerk is 25-30 percent higher than in the push-press and about 50-60 percent higher than in the press.

Push-Press

The push-press is a dynamic movement exercise in which we push the kettlebell from the rack position to a position above the head, using the legs as the main moving force with minimal involvement of the shoulder girdle and arms. It is also a basic exercise for the jerk.

Like the press, the push-press and jerk also begin from the rack position and end with the kettlebell above the head in the lock-out position.

Push-Press

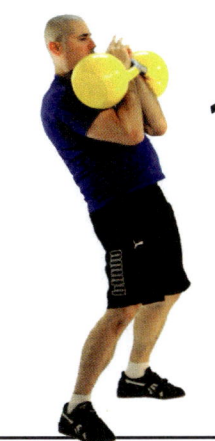 **1** Descend slightly to a front squat (the knee moves forward). While descending, arms maintain contact with the ribs/pelvis.

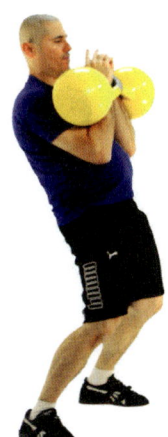 **2** Quick jump on the toes. Leg momentum makes the arm leave the ribs/pelvis and straighten upward.

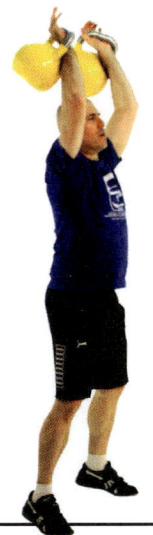 **3** Lower the heels and complete straightening the arm.

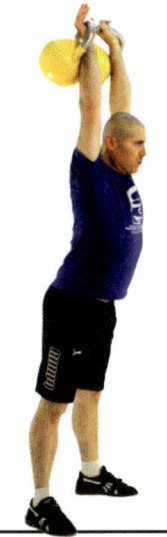 **4** To conclude, the legs are straight and the arms are straight up.

Jerk

The jerk is an explosive movement exercise that lifts the kettlebell from the rack position to above the head, using the jerk movement and a double-dip action of the legs. Shoulders and arms stabilize the kettlebell. As in the press and push-press, the jerk ends with legs straight and arms straight up in the lock-out position.

Jerk

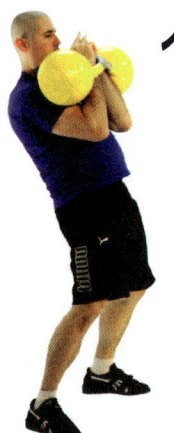 **1** Descend slightly into a front squat. While descending arms maintain contact with the ribs/pelvis.

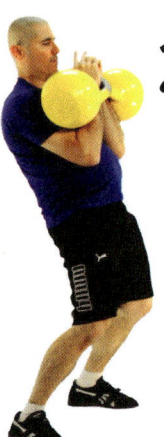 **2** A quick jump on the toes (legs straight) from leg momentum. With help from the chest, arms break contact with the body and straighten at head height.

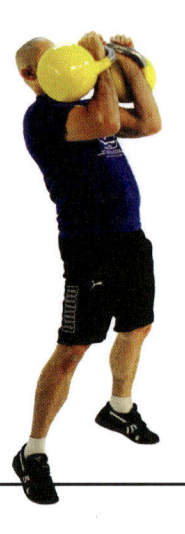

3 Lower the body quickly under the kettlebell (legs slightly bent and arms fully extended).

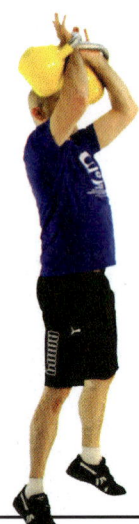

4 Fully extend the legs to erect standing position, arms and legs straight in lock-out position.

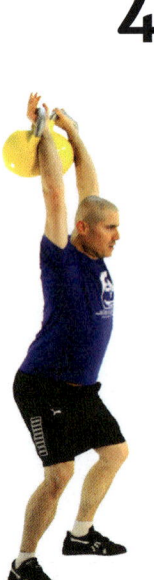

5 End with legs straight and arms straight and fully extended above.

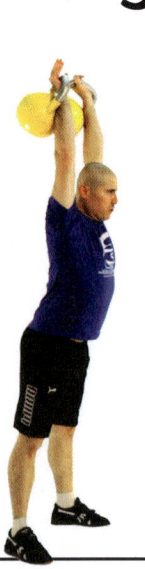

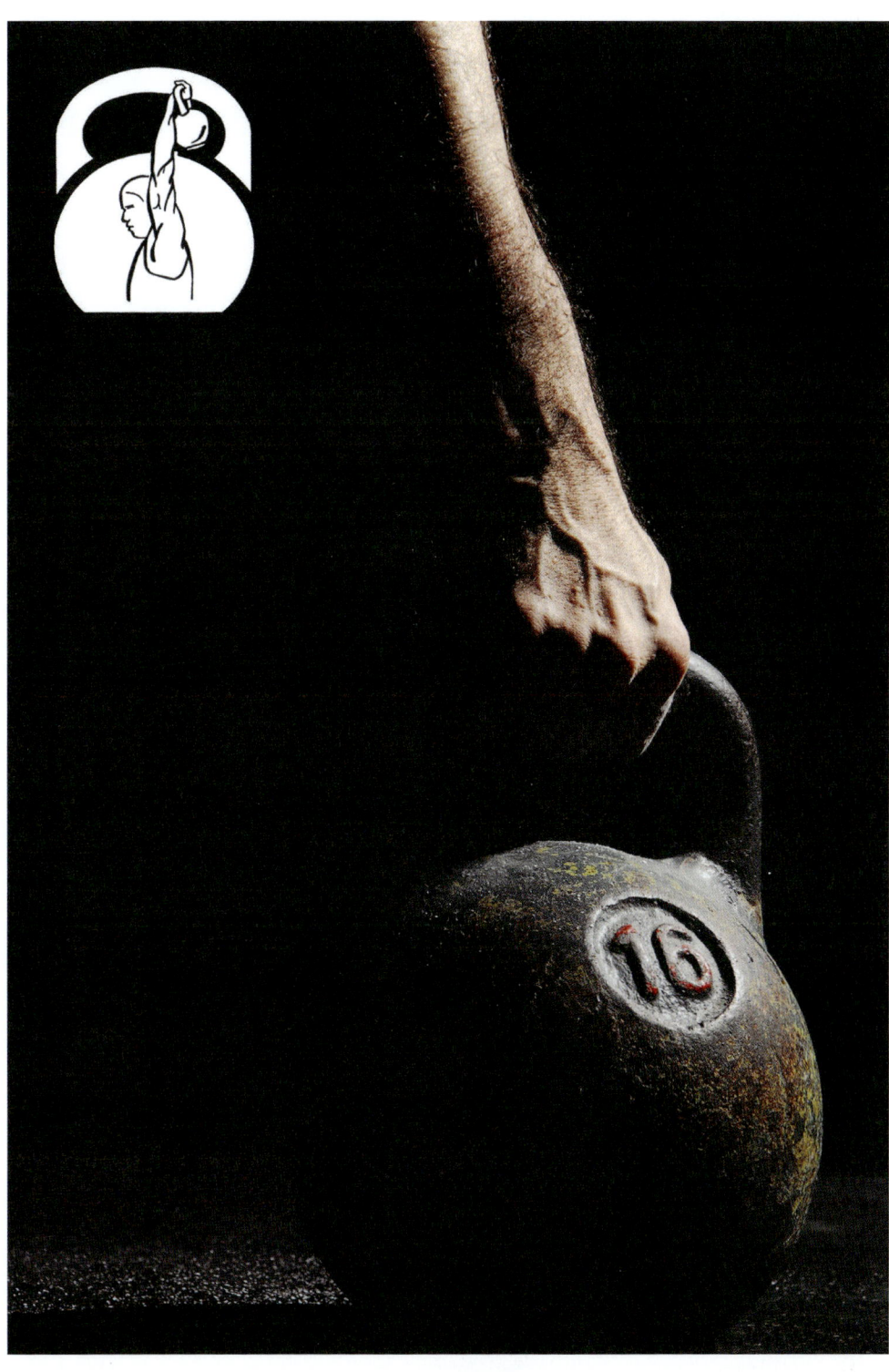

Long cycle

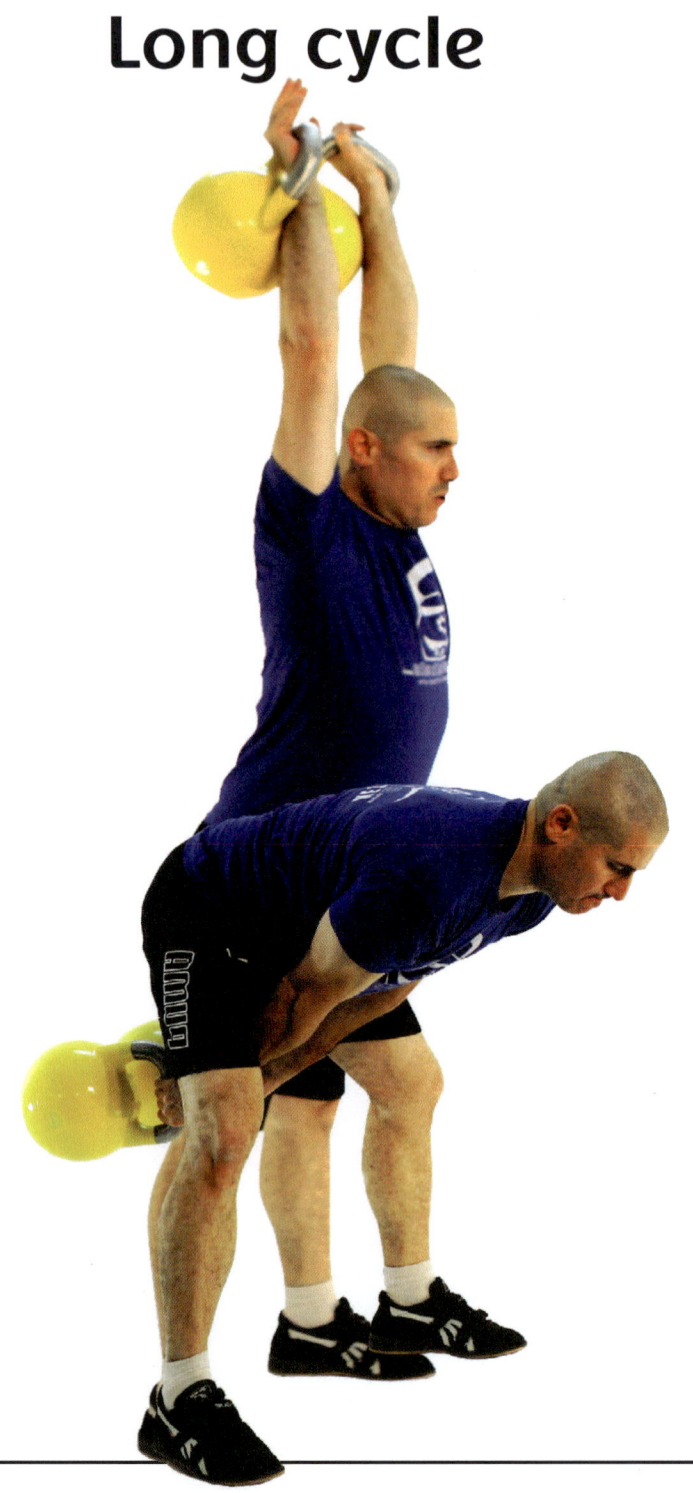

4.6.8 Long Cycle

After we have learned and practiced the clean, rack position and press, we can combine the components into one complex exercise. The long cycle is a dynamic/explosive movement exercise whose aim is to move the kettlebell from between the legs to above the head in two movements. The classic long cycle is comprised of the clean to rack position exercise, and from the rack position to the overhead position through the jerk.

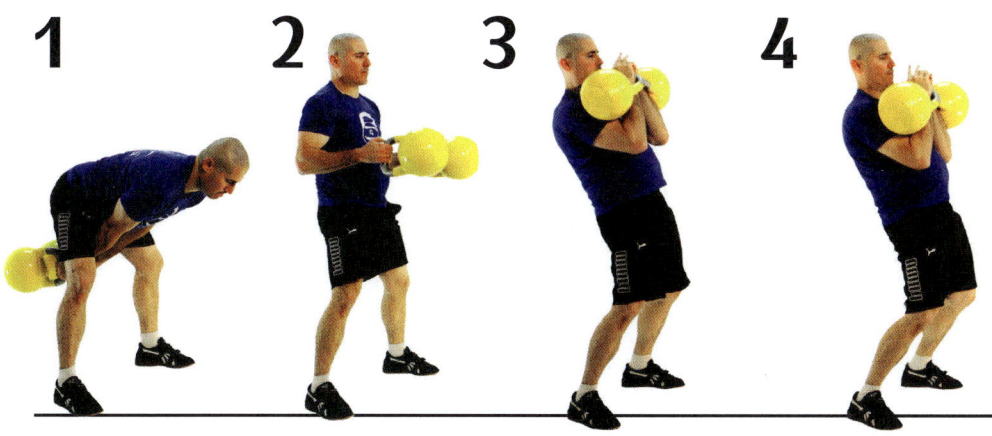

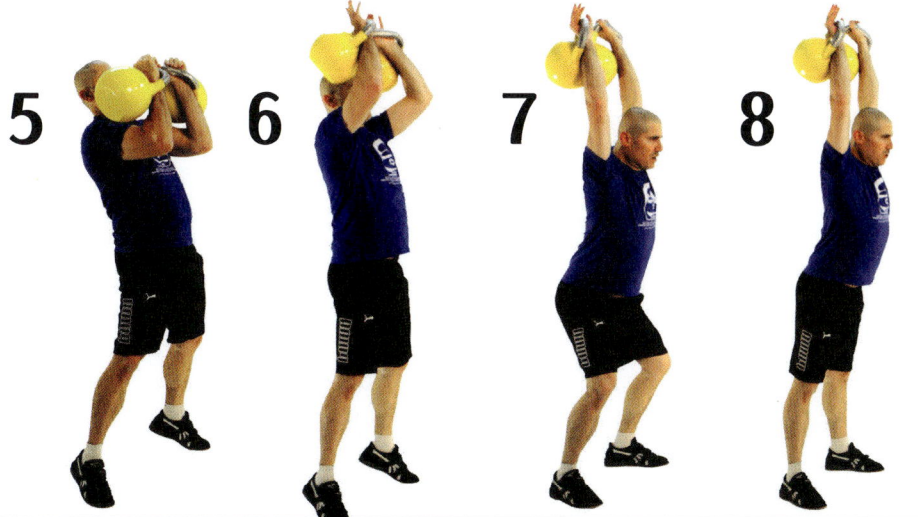

Exercise variations and adaptations:

Long cycle – Press

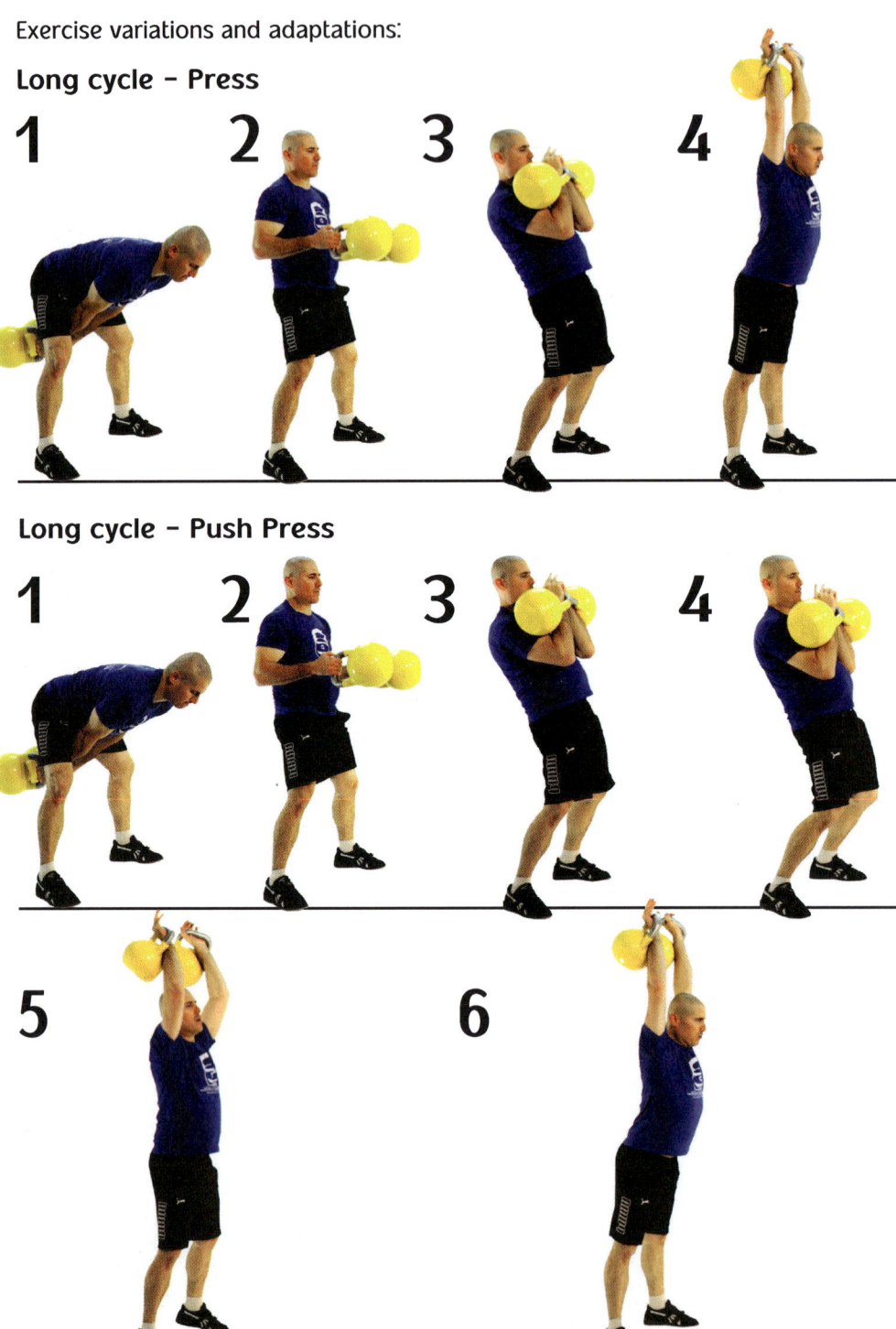

Long cycle – Push Press

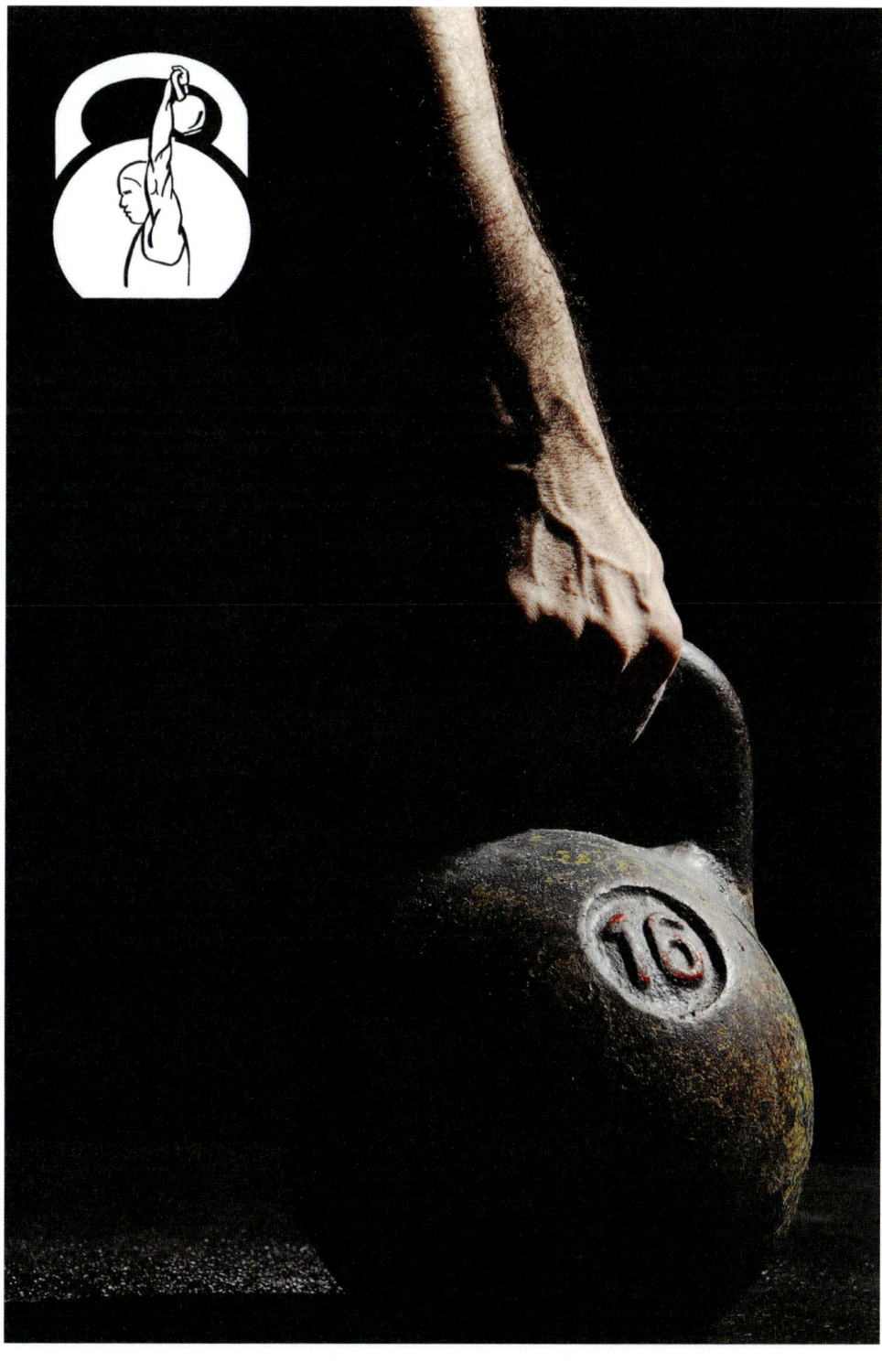

Windmill

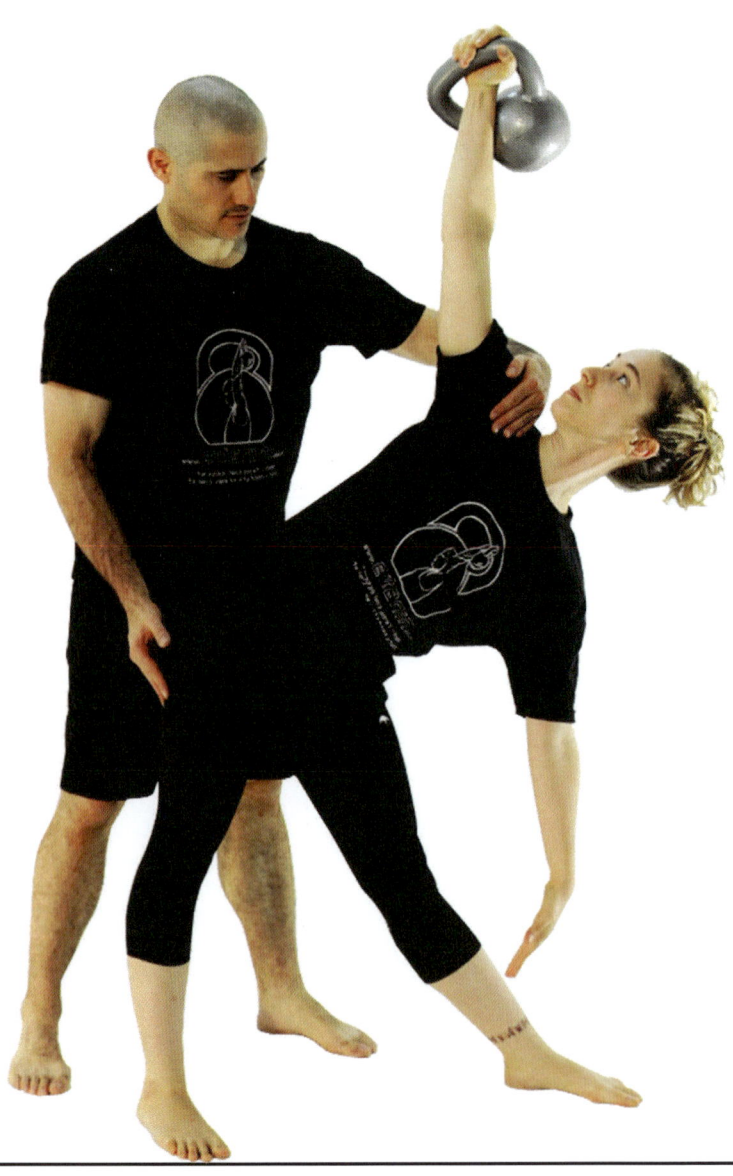

4.6.9 Windmill

The windmill is a basic exercise that is performed in the frontal plane. The windmill teaches us about imbalance between body sides and between the upper and lower parts of the body.

Mobility – the joints that are supposed to move: hip, slight twisting and extension of the thoracic and cervical spine.

Stabilization – the joints that are not supposed to move: foot, ankle, knee, pelvis, lumbar spine, scapula, shoulder, elbow, wrist.

Windmill

Starting position:

Left hand holds the kettlebell up, the free hand is placed on the right thigh. Rotate the feet away from the hand holding the kettlebell.

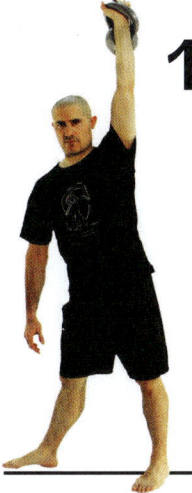

1 While inhaling, push the left hip to the side and push down with the right foot (tilting the pelvis). The left hand holds the kettlebell perpendicular to the ground and the free right hand slides toward the right leg.

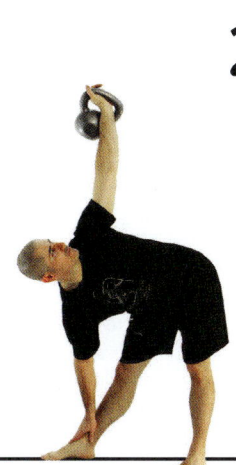

2 While exhaling, maintain the center of the body in balance, push feet against the ground and push the body up again. Do the same on the left side.

Variations of the exercise:

2H Windmill (windmill with two hands)

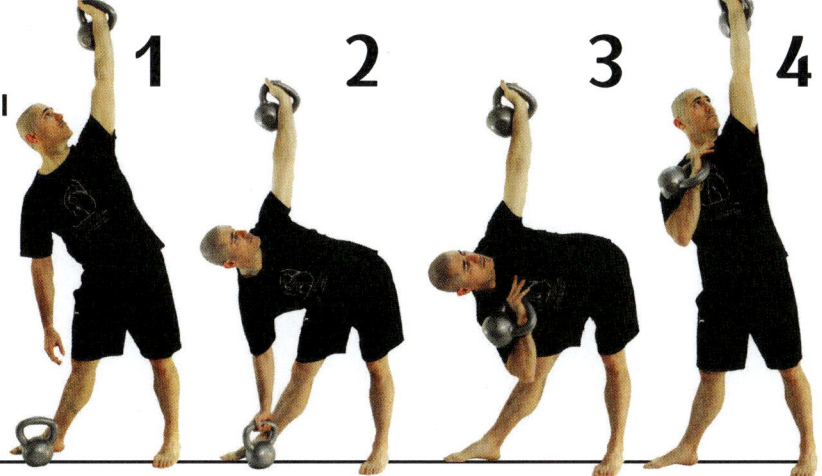

1   **2**   **3**   **4**

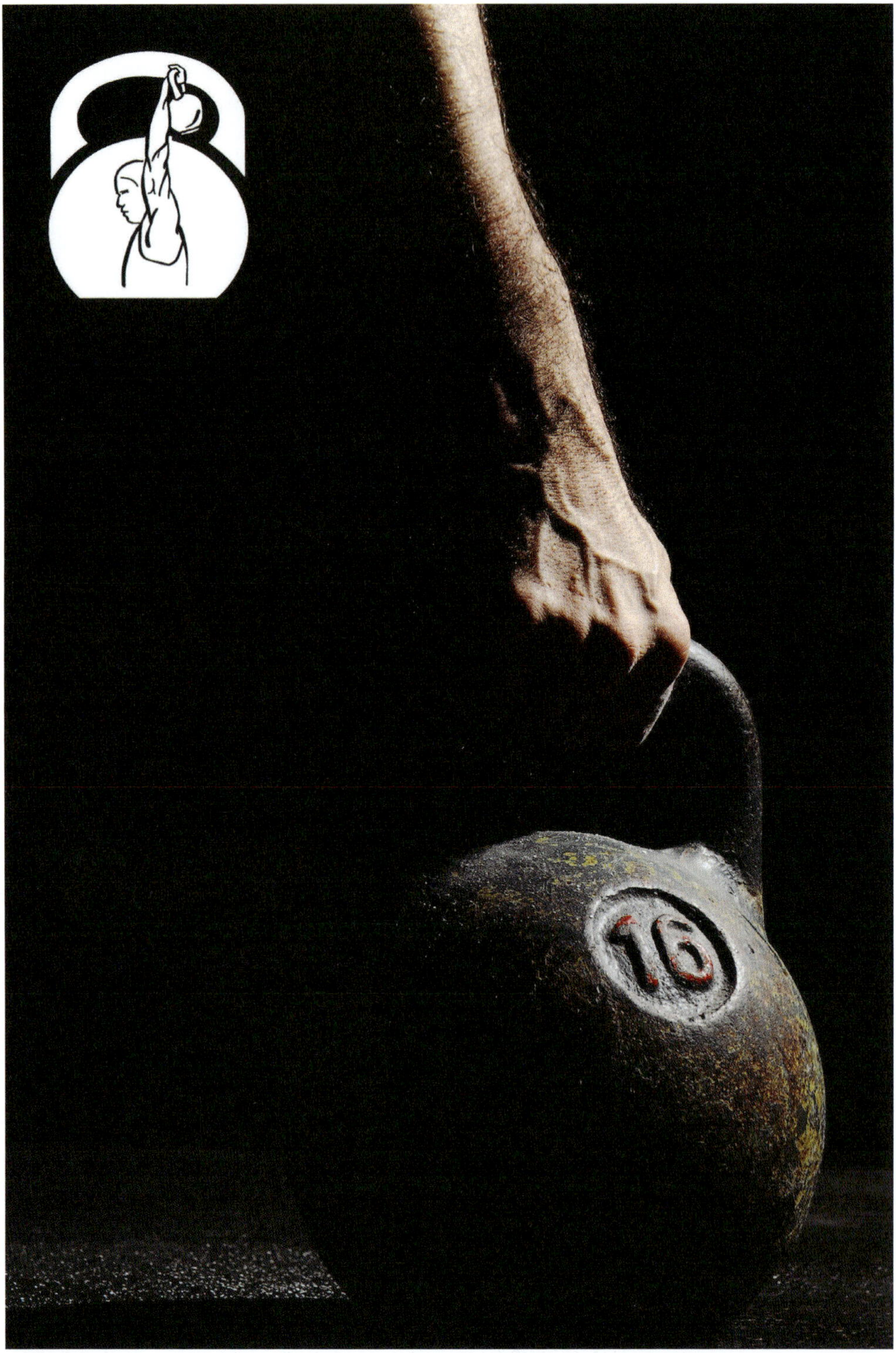

Snatch

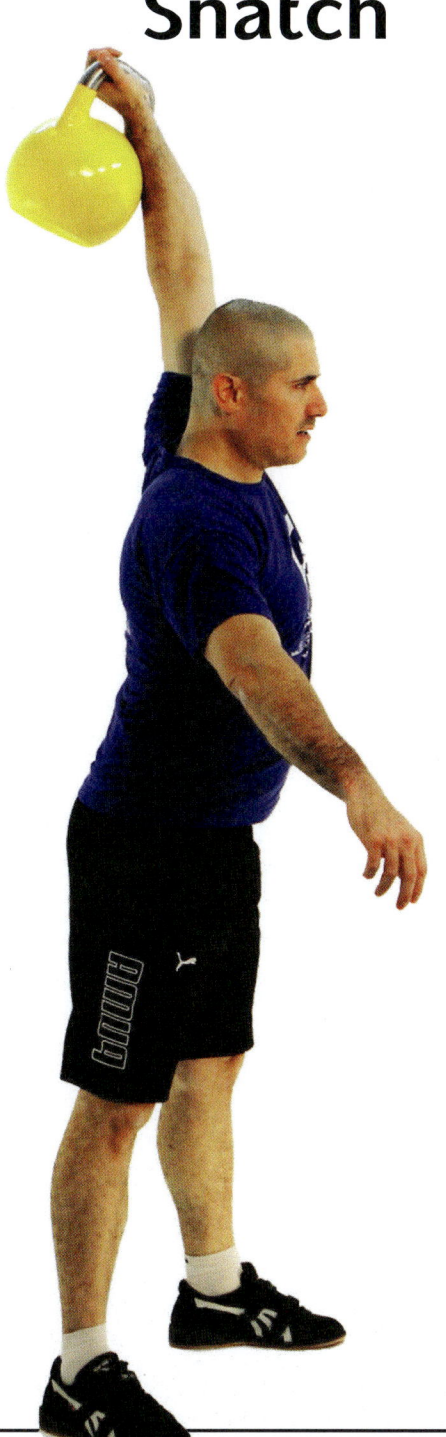

4.6.10 Snatch

Snatch is a dynamic/explosive movement exercise in which the kettlebell is swung from between the legs to above the head in one coordinated movement. Becoming skillful in snatch technique requires a very high level of athletic abilities and skills as well as physical strength.

Preparatory exercise:

High Pull

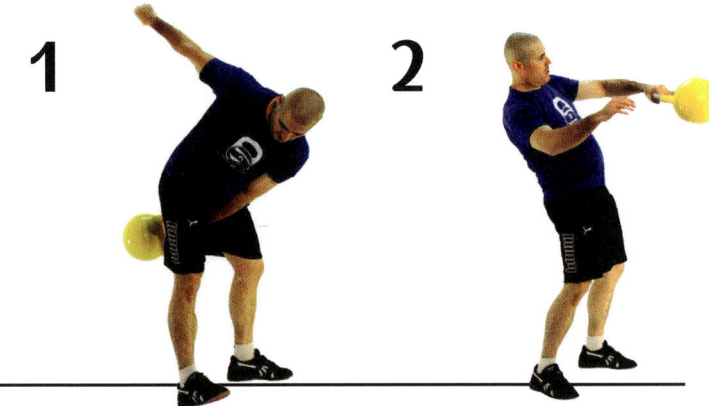

Snatch

Bring the kettlebell to the starting position by snatching it safely (see pages 59)

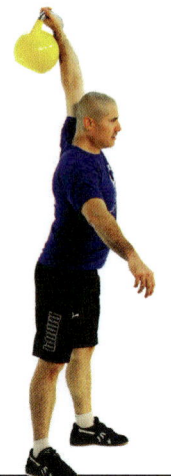

Starting position:
Full extension
(straightening)
of the legs and
left arm straight
in lock-out
position

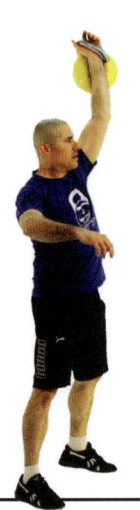

1 Lower the kettlebell -
Tilt the body backward
and let the kettlebell fall
between the legs (as close
as possible to the body,
where the elbow pulls
inward to the center of
the body and the forearm
is perpendicular to the
ground).

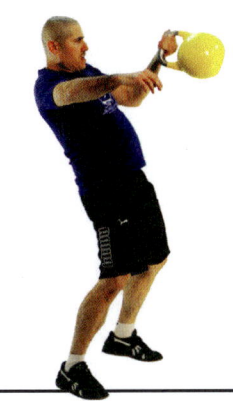 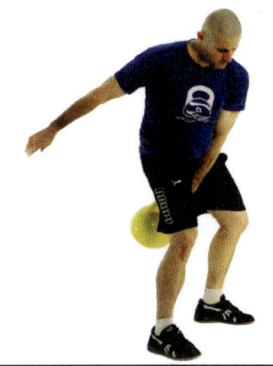 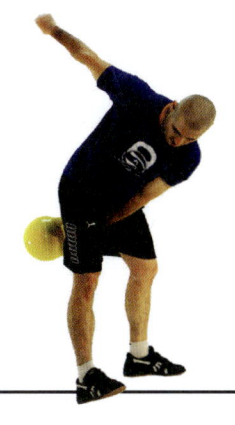

2 Snatch - during the snatch (lifting the hip and the heel on the side of the snatching arm) keep the arm in contact with the ribs/pelvis (moving the pelvis forward and drawing the back to the rear).

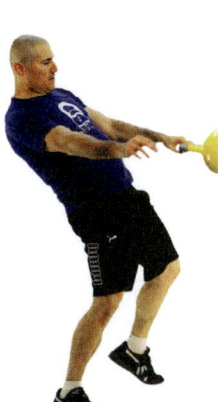

3 Pull - at the end of the upward momentum of the kettlebell, pull the left side and push the right.

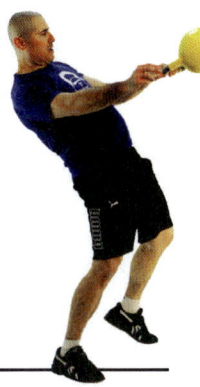

4 Quickly bring the body under the kettlebell.

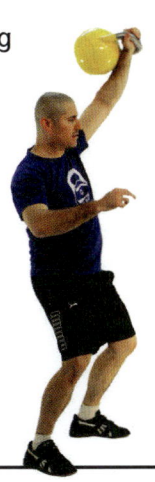 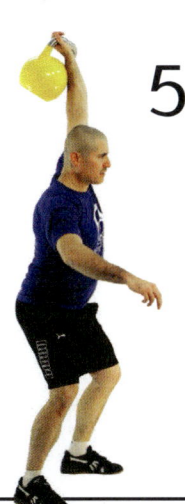

5 Full straightening of the legs to erect standing position. In the final position, legs are straight and the arm is straight in the lock-out position.

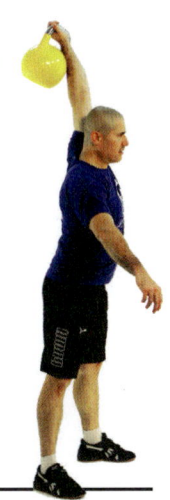

Variation and simplification of the exercise

Half Snatch

The kettlebell is lowered using the half snatch through the rack position.

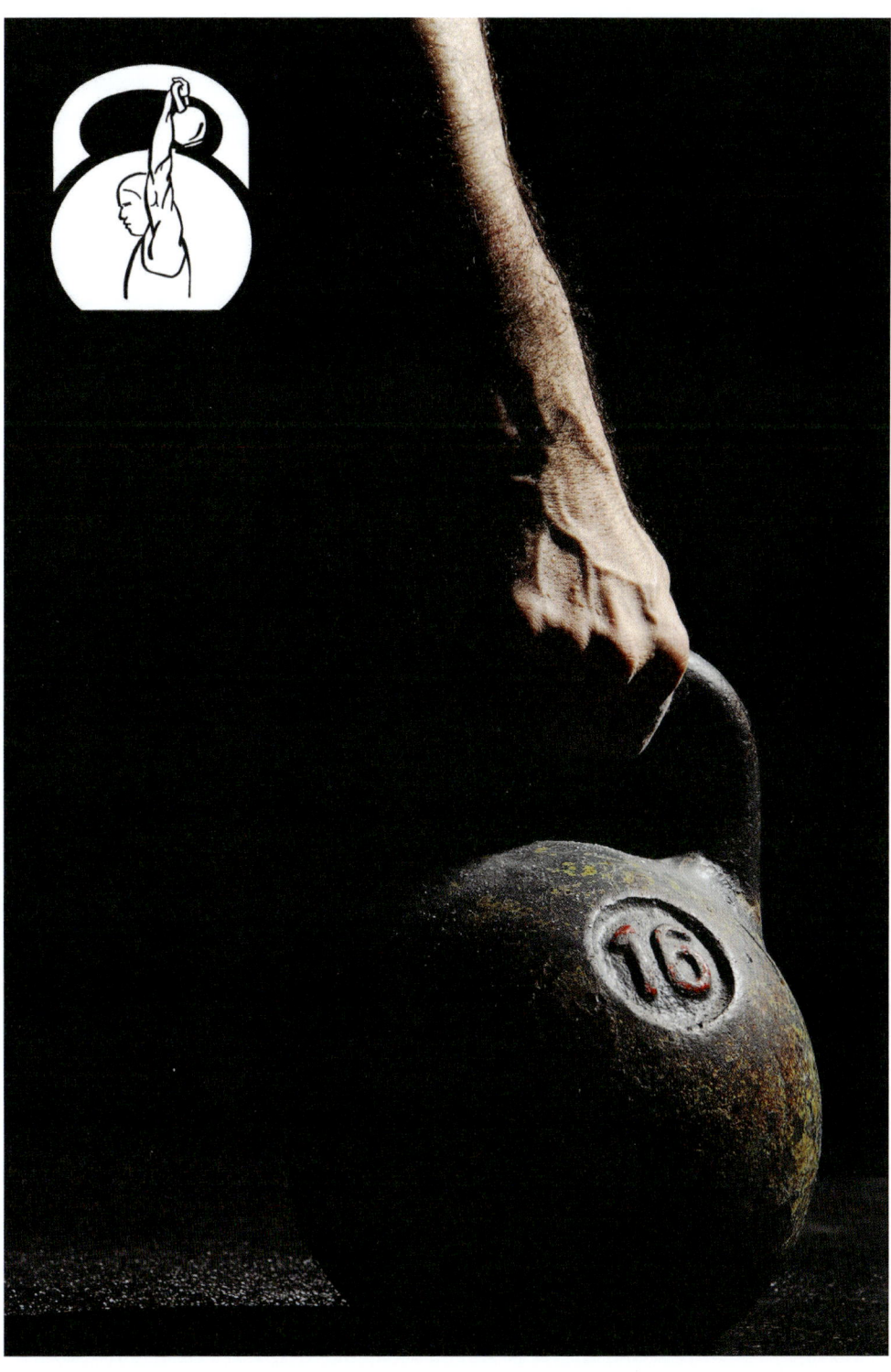

4.6.11 Compilation of exercises:

4.6.11.1 Thrusters

Squat and push the kettlebell in one flow.

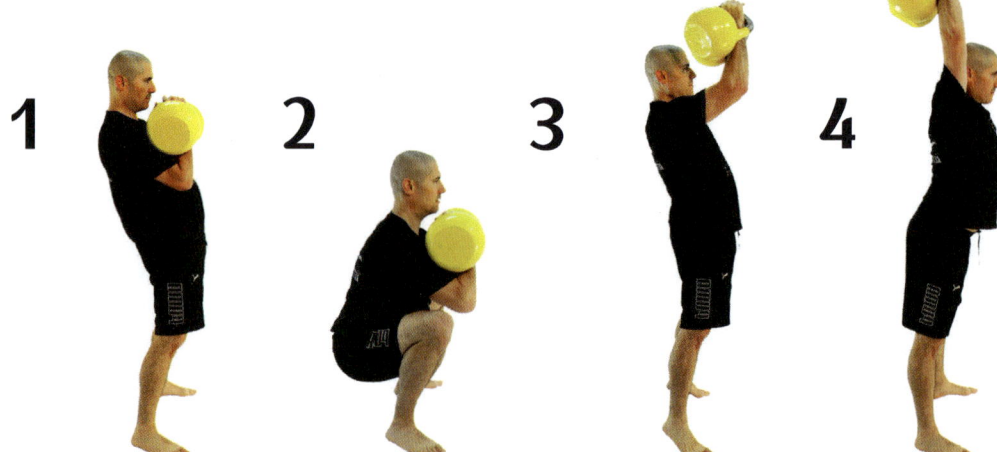

4.6.11.2 Overhead Rotations

Mobility - hip and thoracic spine
stability - lumbar spine

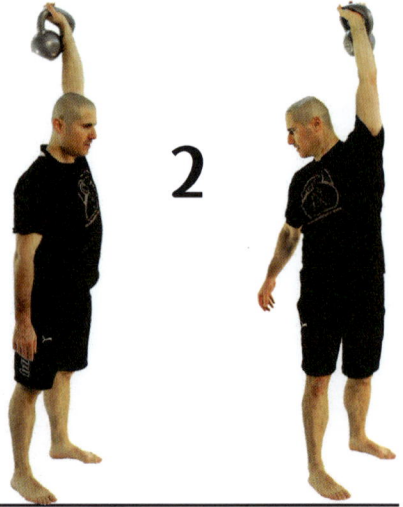

4.6.11.3 Lunge

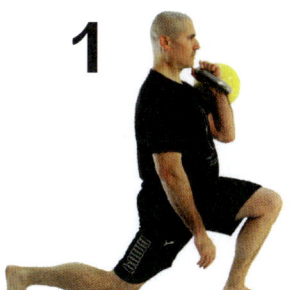
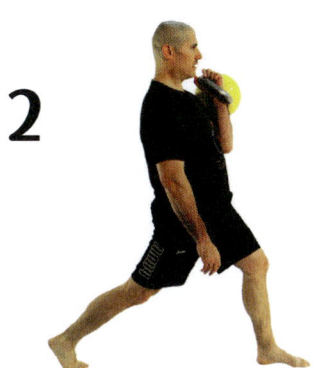

4.6.11.4 Overhead lunge

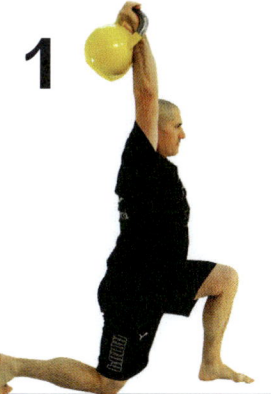
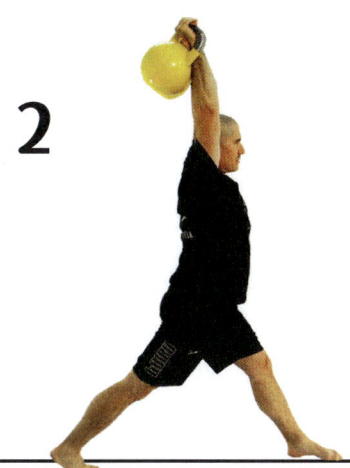

4.6.11.5 Lateral lunge

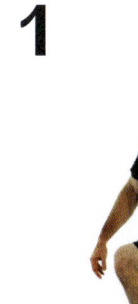
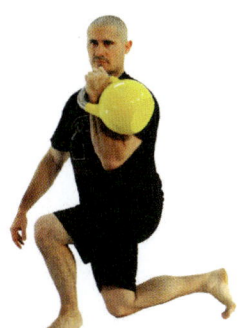
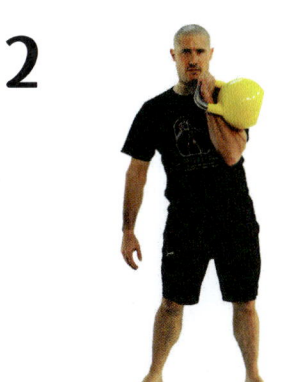

4.6.11.6 Halo

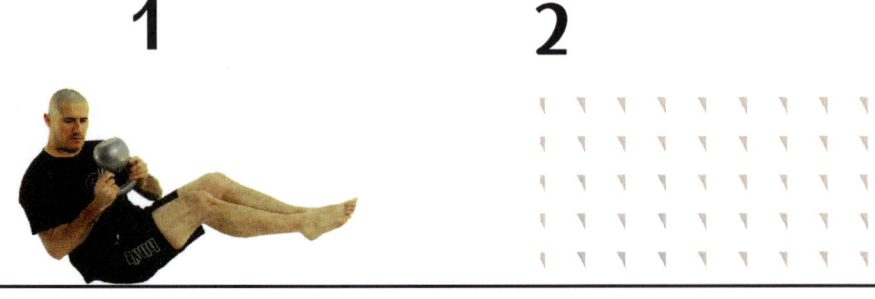

1 **2**

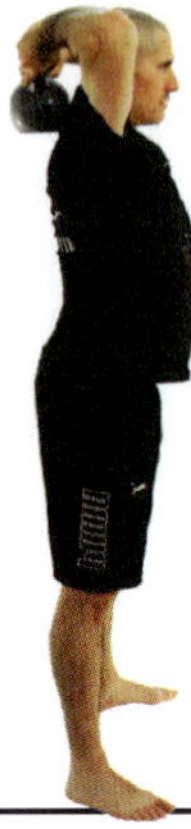

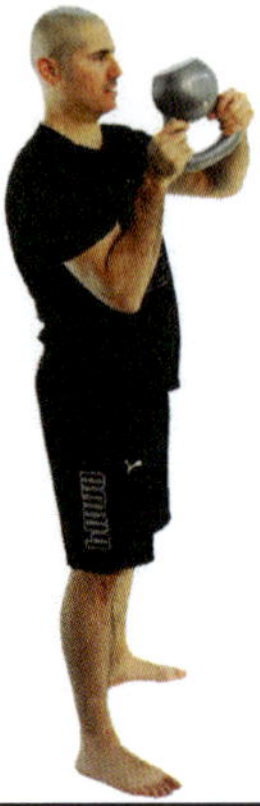

3 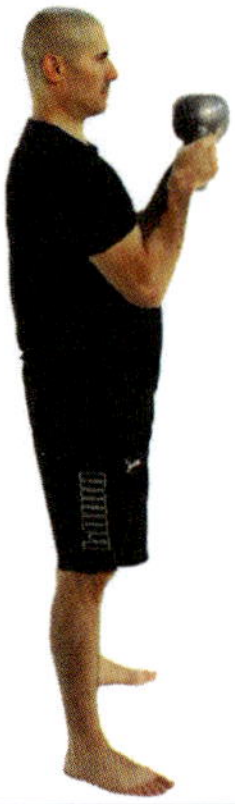 **4**

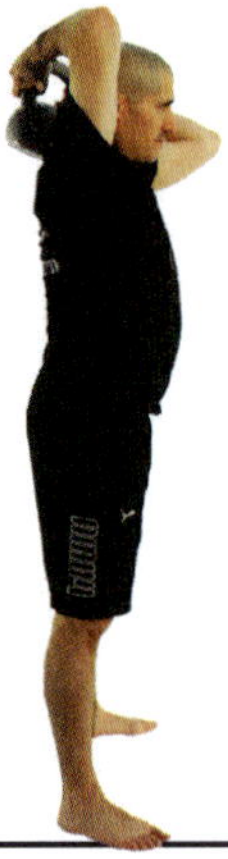

4.6.11.7 Russian twist

Mobility - hip and thoracic spine; stability - lumbar spine

1 **2**

4.6.11.8 Wood chop

Mobility - hip and thoracic spine; stability - lumbar spine

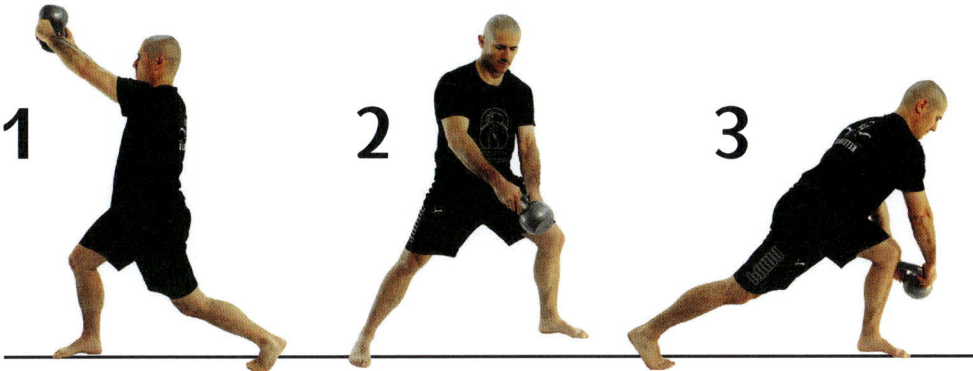

4.6.11.9 Leg lift

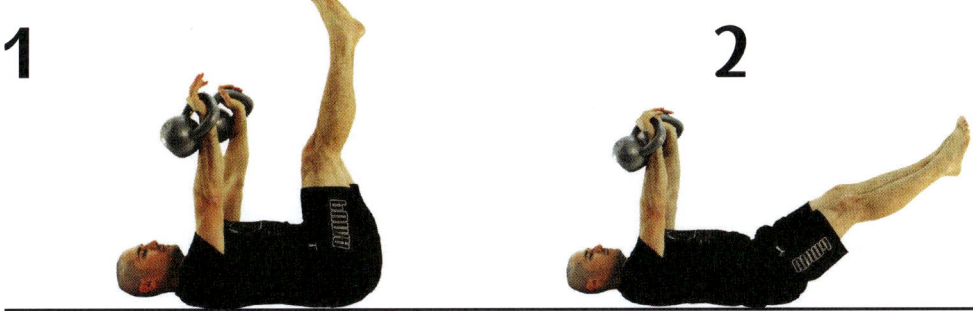

4.6.11.10 Renegade row

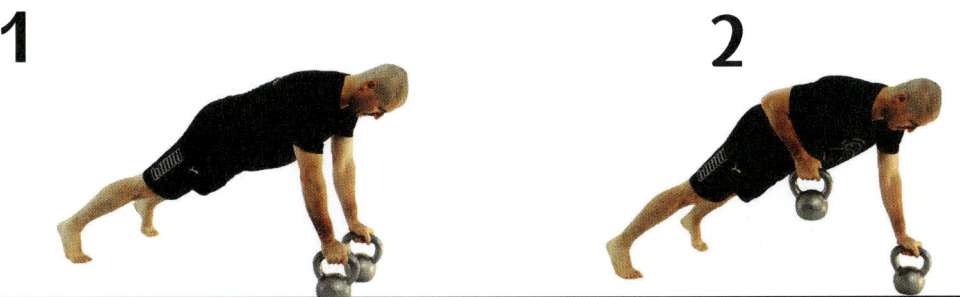

4.6.11.11 Uri Kaduri

1 While exhaling, pull upward

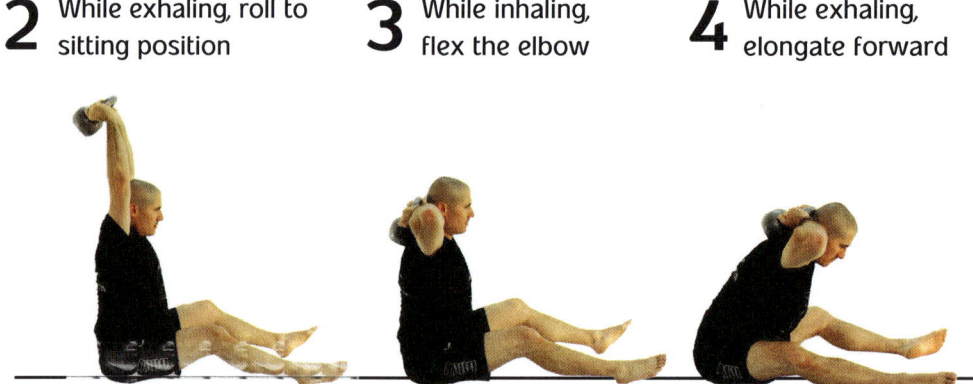

2 While exhaling, roll to sitting position   **3** While inhaling, flex the elbow   **4** While exhaling, elongate forward

5 While inhaling, extend the spine   **6** While exhaling, extend the elbow

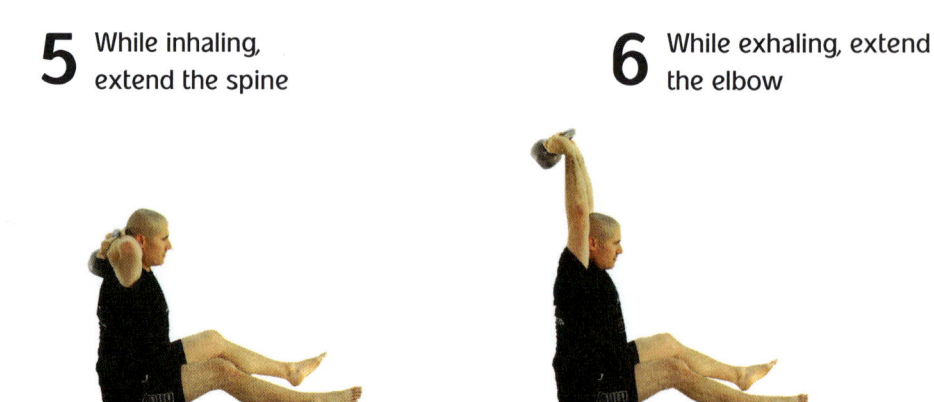

7 While exhaling, roll to supine position

8 While inhaling, return arms to the rear

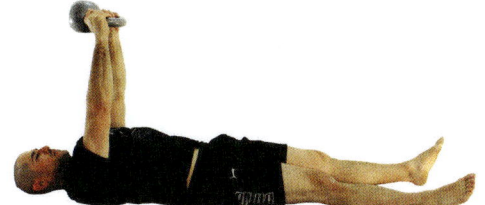
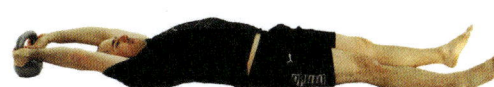

9 While exhaling, roll legs over and beyond the head

10 While exhaling, lower the back

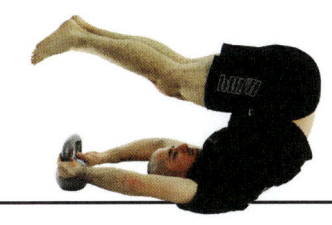
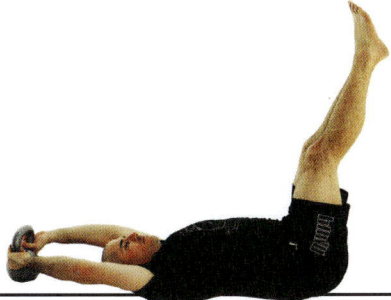

11 While exhaling, lower the legs

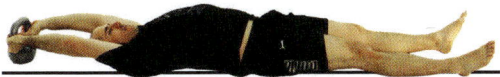

4.6.11.12 Supplementary exercises

The need for supplementary exercises

Just as no one practice method works for everyone, kettlebells also has its limitations. In order to create an effective and more complete and systematic practice, I felt it was necessary to include supplementary exercises to compensate for any shortcomings of kettlebell practice. As noted, we began the practice with mobility on a stiff foam roller to release movement limitations, then moved on to mobility warm-up and practicing basic movement patterns before continuing with the practice itself.

Ring pull / Ring Pull-up

Gym ring - Ring practice is based on body weight exercises using free movement. It offers options for a wide range of exercises adaptable to all levels.

Among the many exercises, an important addition to kettlebell practice is the ring pull. This is an important supplementary exercise for building general strength in the upper part of the body, increasing stability in the shoulder/scapulae and enhancing functional ability, mobility and stability of the scapulae, shoulder girdle and back.

In the exercise pay special attention to stabilizing the scapulae, that is, while pulling down control scapular stability. The rowing exercise can serve as an alternative for exercisers who cannot perform the pull-up exercise.

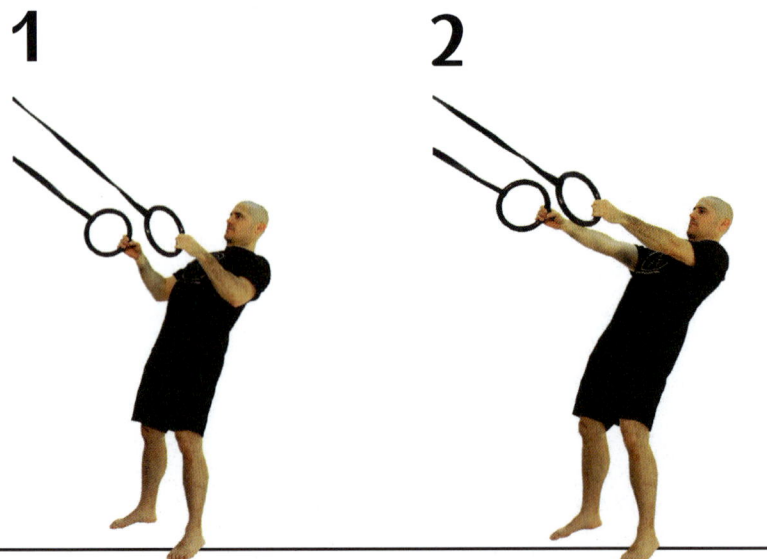

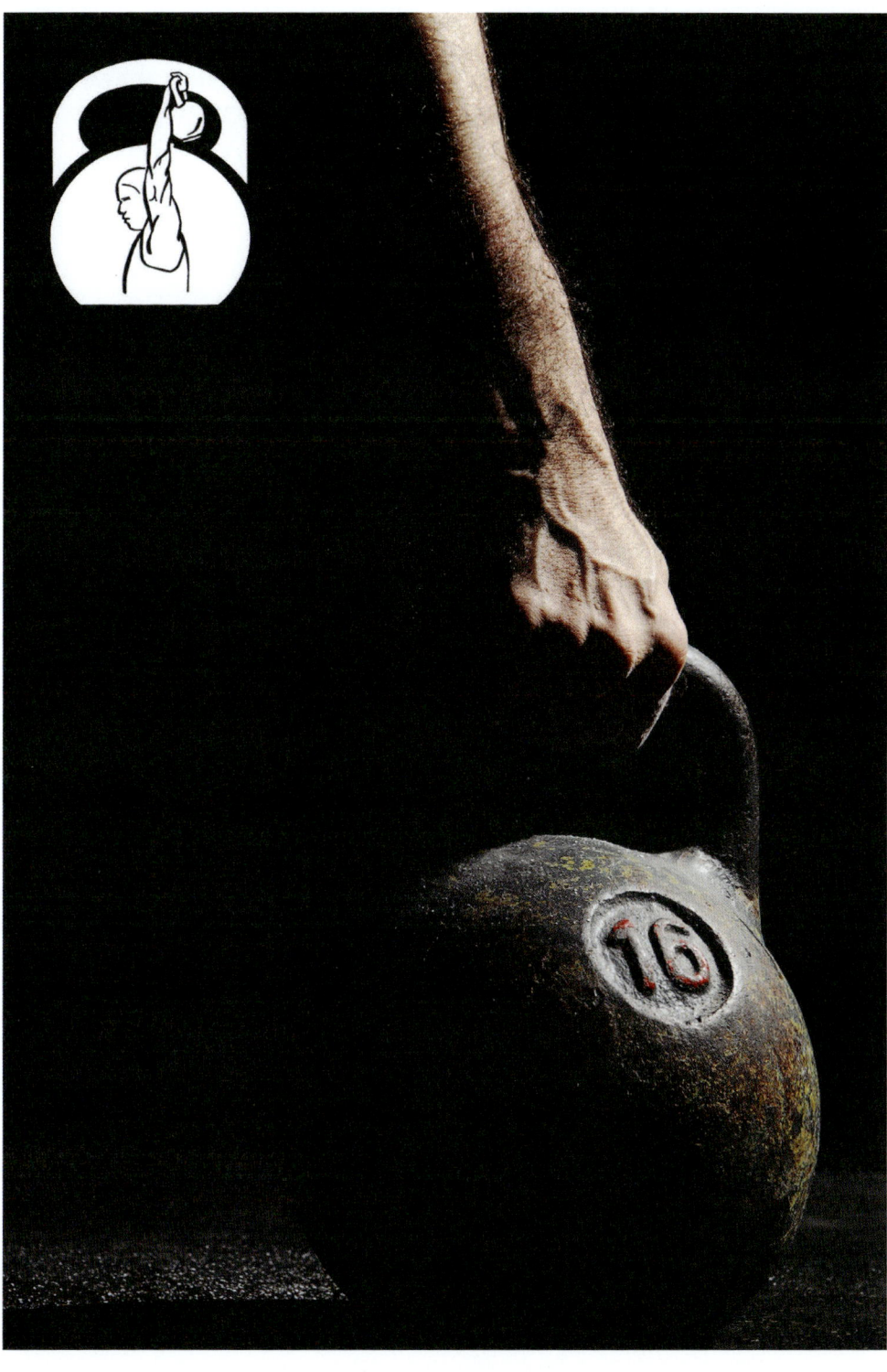

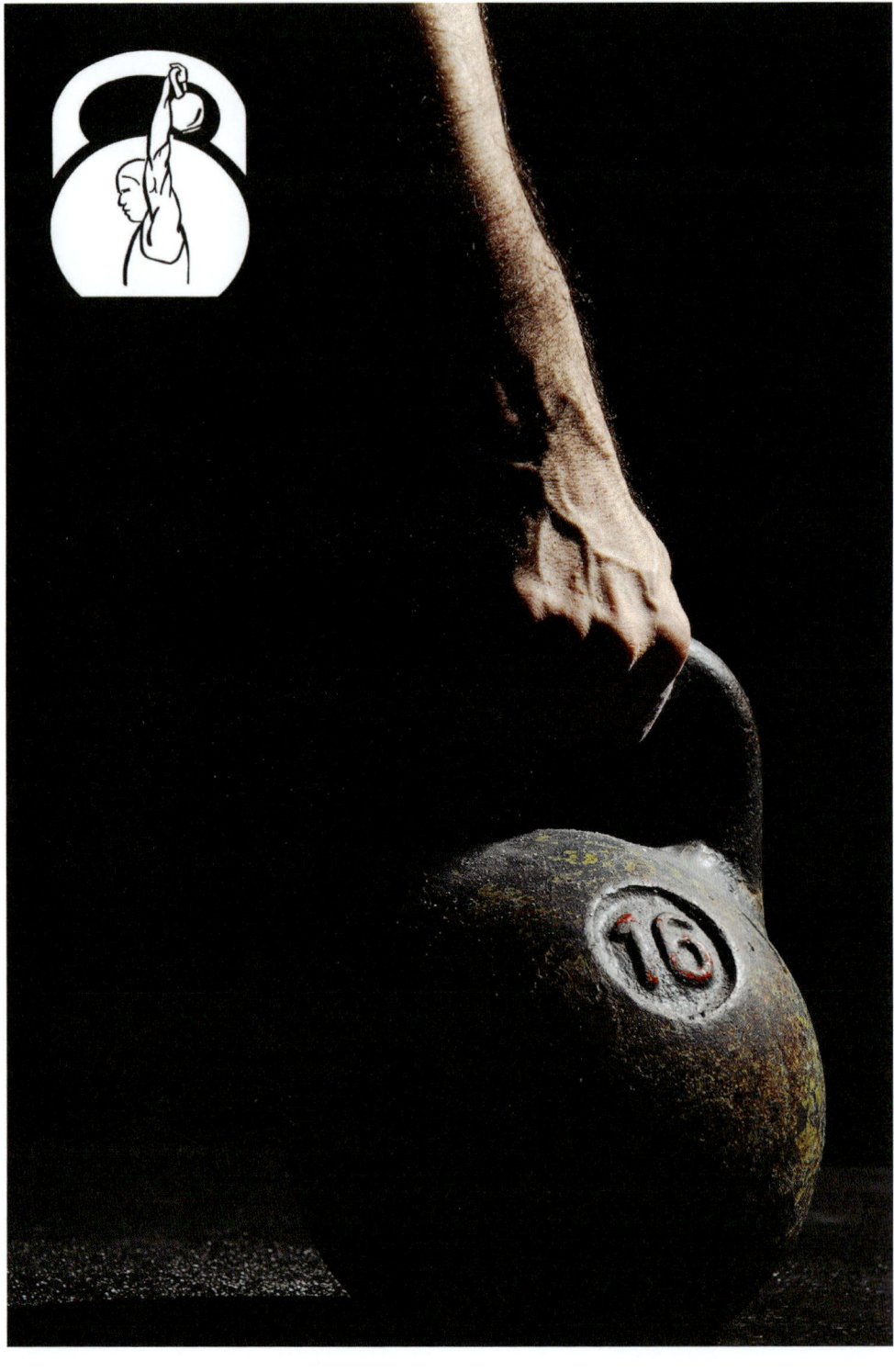

Chapter 5

Program of functional movement practice

- Structure of functional movement practice

- Stages of functional movement practice

- Variables affecting the intensity of movement practice

- A unit of functional movement practice

- The six rules for functional movement practice

- Safety in practice

5. Program of functional movement practice

And the remnant that is escaped of the house of Judah shall
again take root downward, and bear fruit upward.
(Kings II: 19:30)

Growth and development are the products of digging deep and taking root. In order to attain growth in terms of our mobility and skills, we must invest time in developing and deepening the roots, in other words, in our basic abilities.

5.1 Structure of functional movement practice

Functional movement practice teaches us to move our bodies more effectively. As in the martial arts, functional movement practice is a prolonged learning process, where the main emphasis is on technical skill; in other words, learning that will include and practice the movement until it has been absorbed and become automatic, efficient and accurate.

Through functional movement practice we also improve all of the fitness components (basic, complex and psycho-motor). However, technique always precedes physical fitness, both for health - faulty technique may incur injuries - and for functional reasons - faulty technique does not improve functioning and may prevent exercisers from improving it.

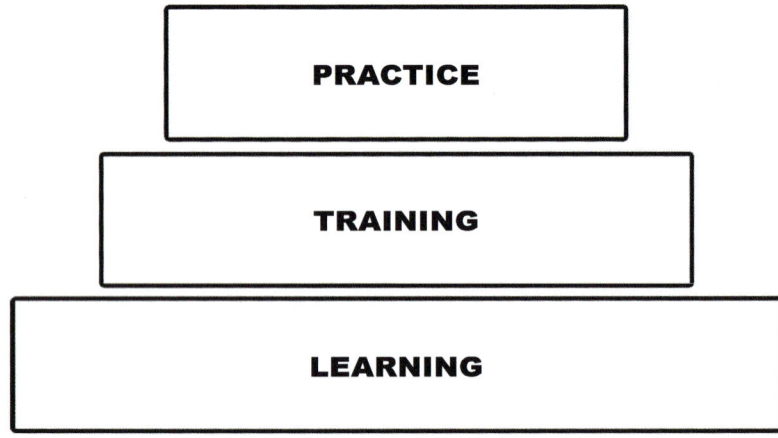

Learning

Understanding the movement, breaking the movement down into parts in order to make learning easier (from the simple to the complex) and practical experience in performing the movement in a comfortable environment (without load or at a slow pace).

Practice

Repeating the movement in simplified conditions (at lower loads, repetition of components) so that the exerciser can internalize the movement and technique correctly and accurately until it becomes automatic.

Training

Strenuous and challenging practice in order to improve the various fitness components and to internalize the correct technique until it becomes automatic.

5.2 Stages of functional movement practice

The following levels of physical requirements are needed for improving mobility in functional movement practice. Progress is gradual, from the easy to the difficult and from the simple to the complex.

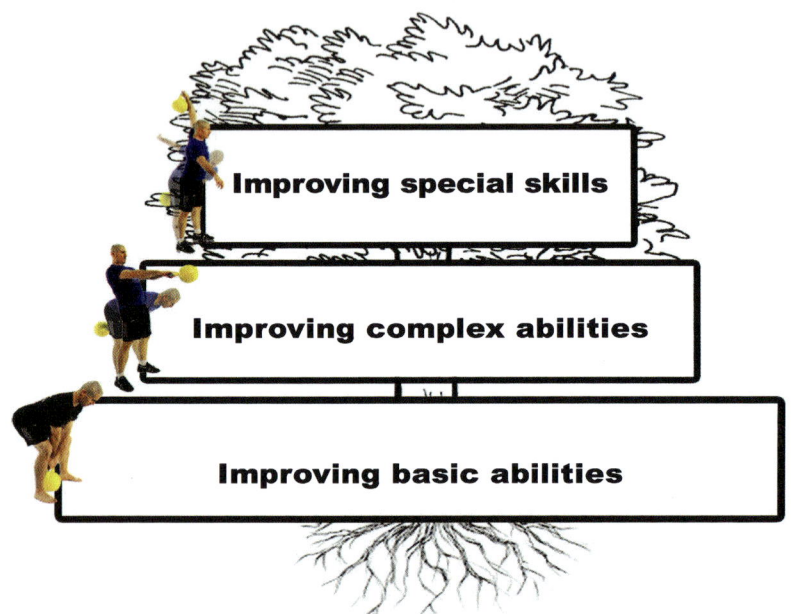

Improving basic abilities

In the first stage we deal with identifying, rehabilitating, preserving (abilities that are not practiced are not preserved) and overcoming weaknesses in basic movement patterns (squat, lift, lunge) with control, without limitation or pain, while softening, expanding ranges of movement and always emphasizing the quality of movement.

Improving complex abilities

After building the base, we connect isolated exercises into complex movements, with an emphasis on mobility, force, loads, precision in movement and efficiency.

Improving special skills

At the top of the pyramid - the focus is on improving technique, skills and special abilities. When the pyramid is built optimally, it is reasonable to assume that exercisers will exhibit good movement ability, as they control their bodies in most positions without limitation, exhibit high level performance and higher than average physical abilities. Where the pyramid is not built optimally, it is reasonable to assume that exercisers will not manifest maximal abilities and performance and are more likely to suffer injuries (lack of strength, flexibility or agility causes limited movement ability).

5.3 Variables affecting the intensity of movement practice

To reach optimal results in practice, we must increase the load. The higher the exerciser's level, the higher the load or stimulus should be.

The practice load or stimulus is usually determined by the following variables:

Rate of repetitions per minute

Each exercise has its own tempo, flow and dynamics. So as not to waste our time counting repetitions, we focus on the quality of movement in each repetition.

For each exercise we will define the duration of the exercise and the number of repetitions required per minute during this time period.

For example: **10 minutes of practice, at a rate of X reps per minute**

Rate of reps/min	Each 3-4 sec	Each 5-6 sec	Each 10 sec
Reps per minute	15-20	10-12	6
10 min practice	150-200	100-120	**60**

Table 4: Rate of repetitions per minute

Minutes per hand

The less often we change hands in snatches, the greater the practice intensity. Changing hands gives the lifting hand a "rest" so that if we lift for one minute with each hand, that is, we switch hands every minute, we are practicing at low intensity. On the other hand, if we lift for five minutes with each hand, that is, we switch hands every five minutes, practice intensity will be high.

Practice with one hand / two hands

Practicing with one hand or two refers to the squat, rack position, clean press, push- press, jerk and long cycle. Practicing with one hand makes learning easier both in terms of load and organizing body position. After learning the technique properly and mastering body organization during the practice, it is possible to increase exercise intensity by working with two kettlebells.

Practice load or duration

The practice load or duration must be such that the technique is maintained and the load is high enough to ensure improvement in performance.

Extending practice time duration

Practice time (individual exercise, cyclical exercise or exercise in one flow) is usually ten minutes long. Gradually, as the exerciser progresses, practice duration can be increased.

Kettlebell weight

For the body to respond positively and to improve (and prevent injuries!), practice loads, increases in complexity and effort should be moderate and gradual, from the easy to the difficult, and from the simple to the complex.

For example – data for the one-handed Clean exercise:

Duration: 4 minutes

Reps per minute: 6 (1 every 10 seconds)

Minutes per hand: 1 (switch hands each minute)

Kettlebell weight: 12 kg

Variables that can affect the level of exercise difficulty:

Variable	Rate of reps per minute	Minutes per hand	Exercise duration	Weight	Hands
Rate of reps per minute	5	1	4 min	12 kg	One
Switch hands per minute	10	2	4 min	12 kg	One
Duration of exercise	10	1	6 min	12 kg	One
Kettlebell weight	10	1	4 min	16 kg	One
Exercise using two hands	10	1	4 min	12 kg	Two

Table 5: Variables that affect intensity of movement practice

It is possible to change one or more exercise variables. To be absolutely clear, **physical fitness** comes first - that is, weight or complexity should not be increased before the exercise is performed with optimal technique.

5.4 A unit of functional movement practice

A unit of practice should include exercises from all the movement patterns (squat, lift, lunge, push, pull, twist and walk/run).

Number of practices per week: 3-5 per week

Practice time: 10-30 minutes

Preparation:

Release movement limitations through mobilization on a stiff foam roller.

Movement warm-up with an emphasis on improving ranges of movement, removing movement limiting factors and increasing awareness.

Practice:

Practice special components, coordination, improving and internalizing technique. Improve mobility and fitness components.

Release:

Improve weak components, release and relaxation.

5.5 The six rules for functional movement practice

1. Hard work

"Hard – that means possible." (Zeev Jabotinsky)

The secret to success in practice, as in life itself, is hard work and determination, with no shortcuts and no discounts. We can only control how much effort we invest, and that is what determines whether we succeed or not.

2. Practice without pain

When pain develops during practice (in contrast to pain from effort or difficulty), the practice must be stopped. We can continue only after identifying the source of the pain and removing the limiting cause.

3. Technique before physical fitness

One of the objectives of practice is to learn movements and skills and to internalize the correct technique until it becomes almost automatic. Strenuous and challenging practice intended only to improve fitness components may lead to exhaustion, which will often cause a decline in movement and functional quality. Practicing improper technique actually ingrains faulty movement patterns, the consequences of which are injuries and less chance of attaining optimal movement patterns.

4. There's no such thing perfect practice. Practice makes perfect

The exercise itself is not the aim of the practice. Consistent and systematic practice slowly leads the exerciser to perfection.

5. Systematic practice

Progress in practice is measured in terms of months and years, and the objective is to improve techniques, skills and movement ability while avoiding wear and tear and injuries. Practice should be moderate and adapted to personal abilities; it should progress gradually, constantly and methodically, both in terms of exercise load and complexity.

6. Simplicity

Simplicity applies to many components and represents the essence of practice. Through systematic practice, complex movements and exercises become simple. They flow naturally and almost without effort. By attaining simplicity, we reveal the quality of our movement.

5.6 Safety in practice

Safety is an integral part of our practice. We must understand the functioning of the body in order to identify movement weaknesses and strong points and to remove elements that limit or endanger us. In practice, as in life, there is no substitute for thought and common sense (your present condition and the practice environment...). The most important rule of practice is:

> **"Last act, but first Think"** – Think before you act
> (Rabbi Shlomo Alkabetz)

Chapter 6

Practice programs

- Suggestions and examples of circuit training and practice in one flow

- Practice programs

6.1 Suggestions and examples of circuit training and practice in one flow

Circuit training ➕

Circuit training is composed of a series of exercises performed one after the other, where **each exercise stands alone, and exercisers move from station to station according to a time schedule**. For example: we perform 60 seconds of Clean, followed immediately, with no rest, by 60 seconds of Press. This sequence is considered one cycle, which we repeat X times.

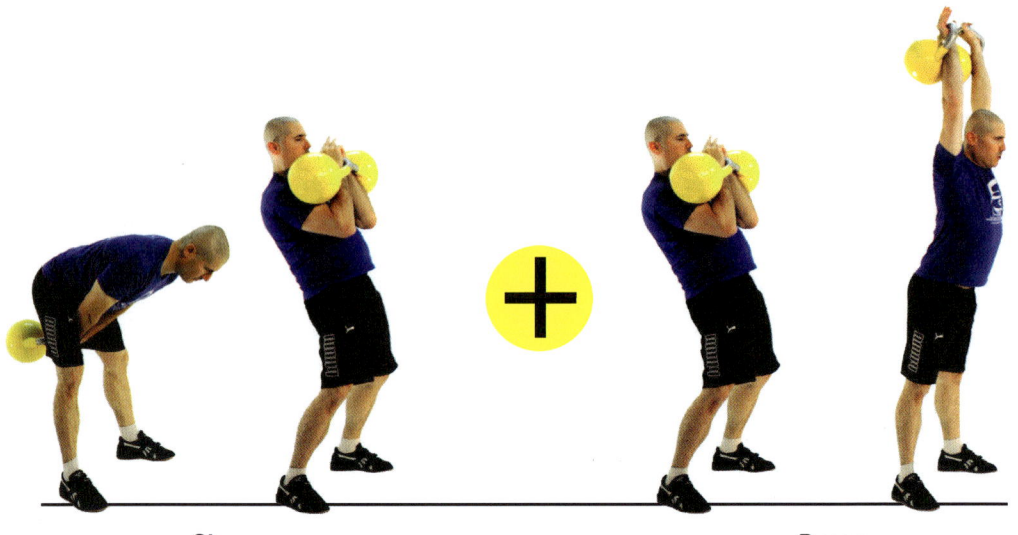

Clean   Press

Suggestions and examples of circuit training ➕

Circuit training No. 1: Good morning + Goblet squats
Circuit training No. 2: Dead-lift + Swing
Circuit training No. 3: Swing + Get up
Circuit training No. 4: Swing + Squat
Circuit training No. 5: Overhead squat + Windmill
Circuit training No. 6: Thrusters + Snatch + Jerk + Long cycle

Practice in one flow ❯

This is a series of exercises performed one after the other. **The exercises flow one into the other, and exercisers switch from one exercise to the next after one repetition.** For example: Long cycle - we perform one repetition of Clean, followed by one of Press. This sequence is considered one circuit which we repeat X times.

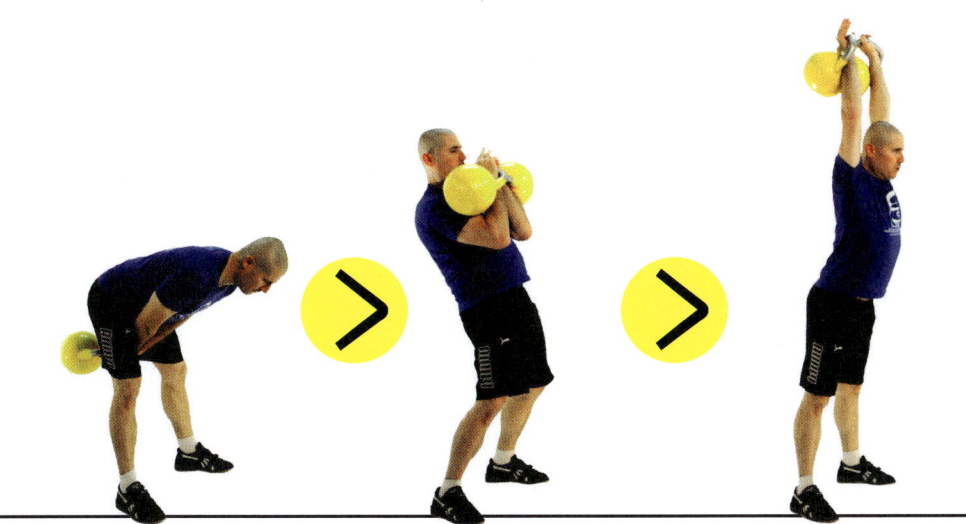

Long cycle

Suggestions and examples of practice in one flow: ❯

Flow No. 1: Get up > Windmill
Flow No. 2: Long cycle
Flow No. 3: Thrusters
Flow No. 4: Clean > Squat > Press
Flow No. 5: Swing > Clean > Squat > Press > Windmill > Get up
Flow No. 6: Swing > Clean > High pull > Snatch

6.1.1 15-minute practice program

An introductory program intended for independent daily practice for beginning exercisers.

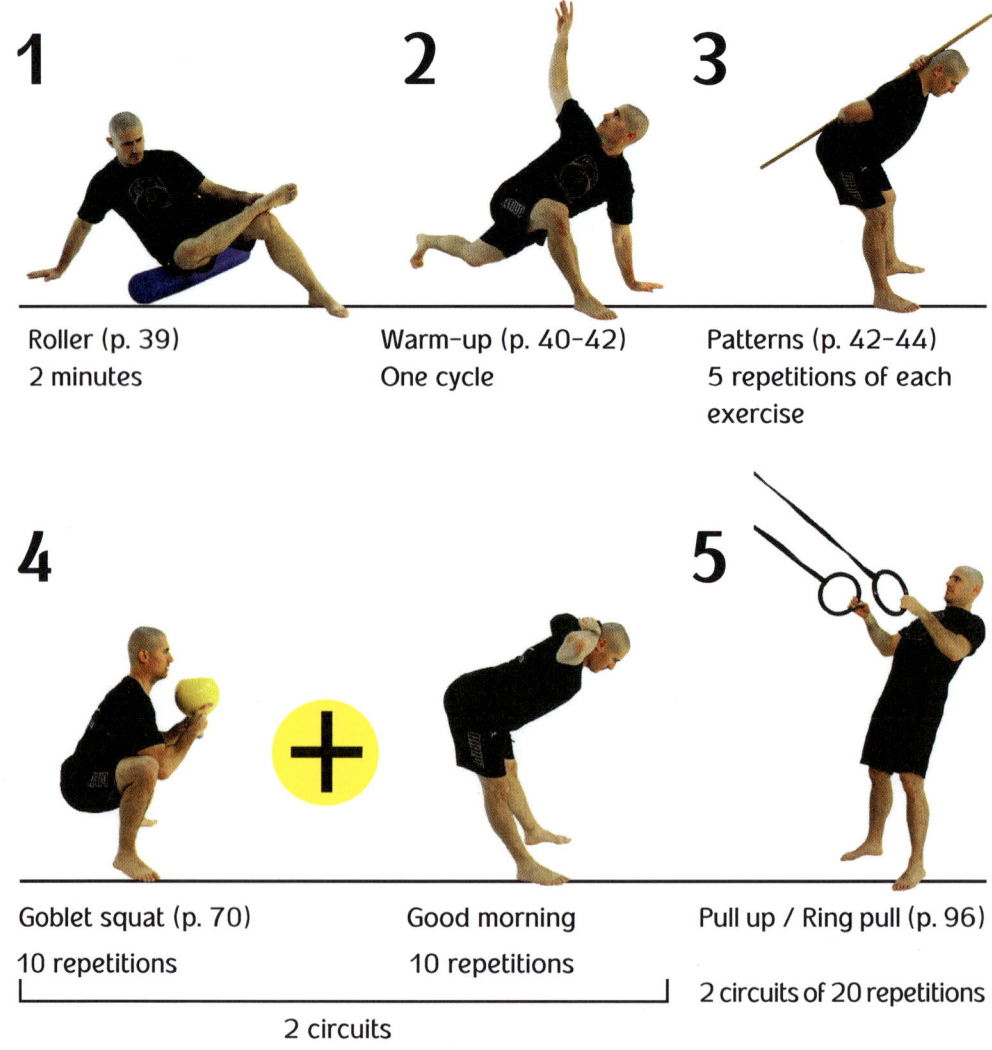

1 Roller (p. 39)
2 minutes

2 Warm-up (p. 40-42)
One cycle

3 Patterns (p. 42-44)
5 repetitions of each exercise

4 Goblet squat (p. 70)
10 repetitions

Good morning
10 repetitions

2 circuits

5 Pull up / Ring pull (p. 96)
2 circuits of 20 repetitions

6.1.2 15-minute practice program

The program is intended for independent daily practice.
The practice is suitable for beginning exercisers who have had basic instruction.

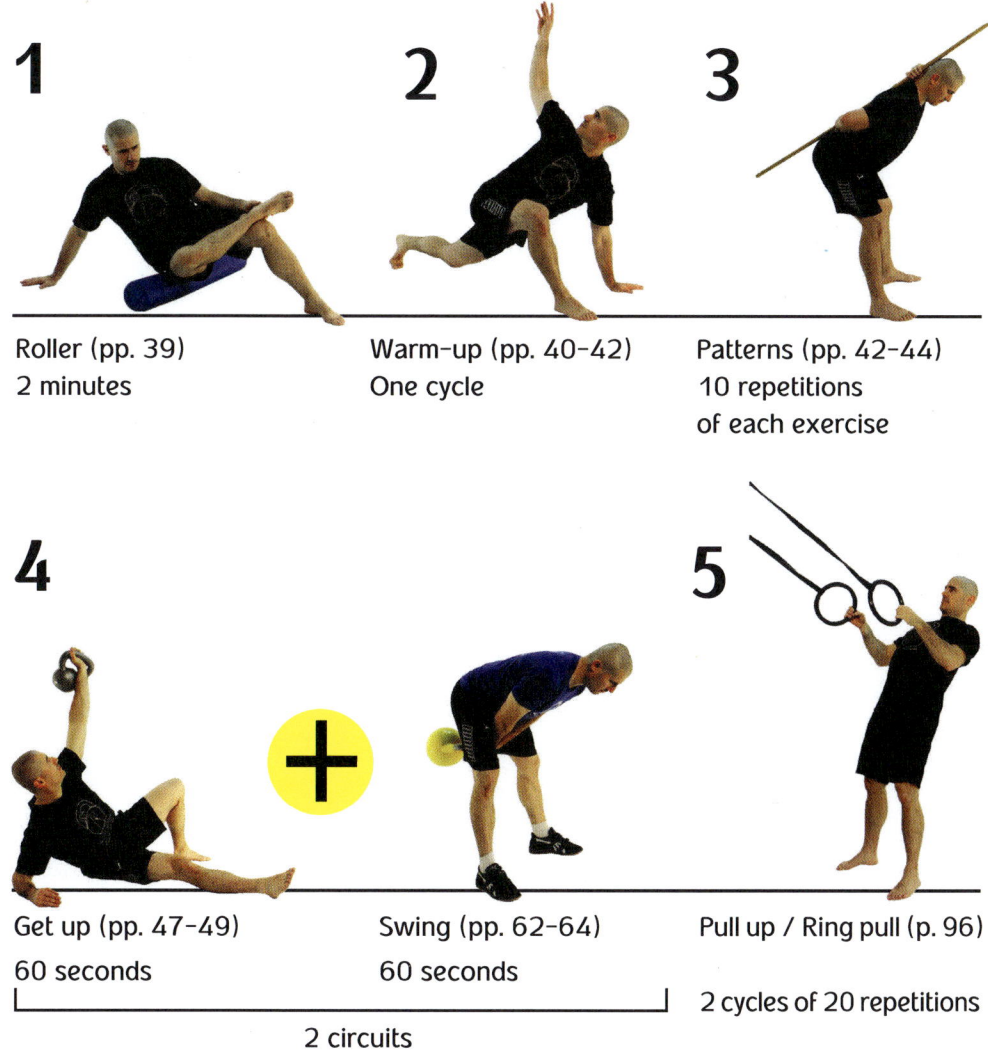

1 Roller (pp. 39)
2 minutes

2 Warm-up (pp. 40-42)
One cycle

3 Patterns (pp. 42-44)
10 repetitions
of each exercise

4 Get up (pp. 47-49)
60 seconds

Swing (pp. 62-64)
60 seconds

5 Pull up / Ring pull (p. 96)

2 cycles of 20 repetitions

2 circuits

6.1.3 30-minute practice program

The program is intended for independent daily practice.
The practice is suitable for exercisers of all levels who have had basic instruction.

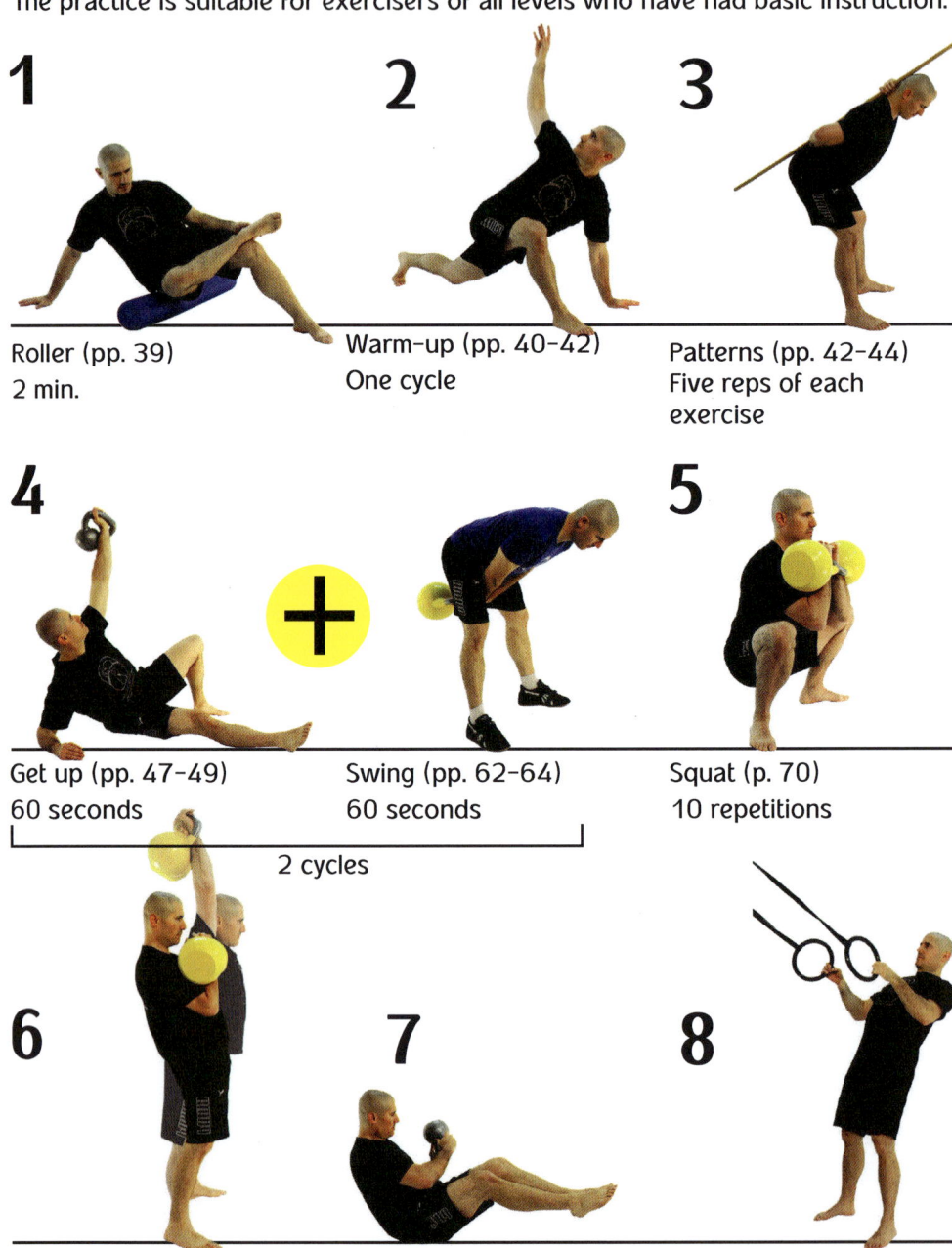

1

Roller (pp. 39)
2 min.

2

Warm-up (pp. 40–42)
One cycle

3

Patterns (pp. 42–44)
Five reps of each
exercise

4

Get up (pp. 47–49)
60 seconds

Swing (pp. 62–64)
60 seconds

2 cycles

5

Squat (p. 70)
10 repetitions

6

Press (pp. 73–76)
2 cycles of 2 min
with each hand

7

Russian twist (p. 92)
2 cycles of 20 repetitions

8

Pull up / Ring pull (p. 96)
2 cycles of 20 repetitions

6.1.4 30-minute practice program

The program is intended for independent daily practice.
The practice is suitable for exercisers at all levels who have had basic instruction.

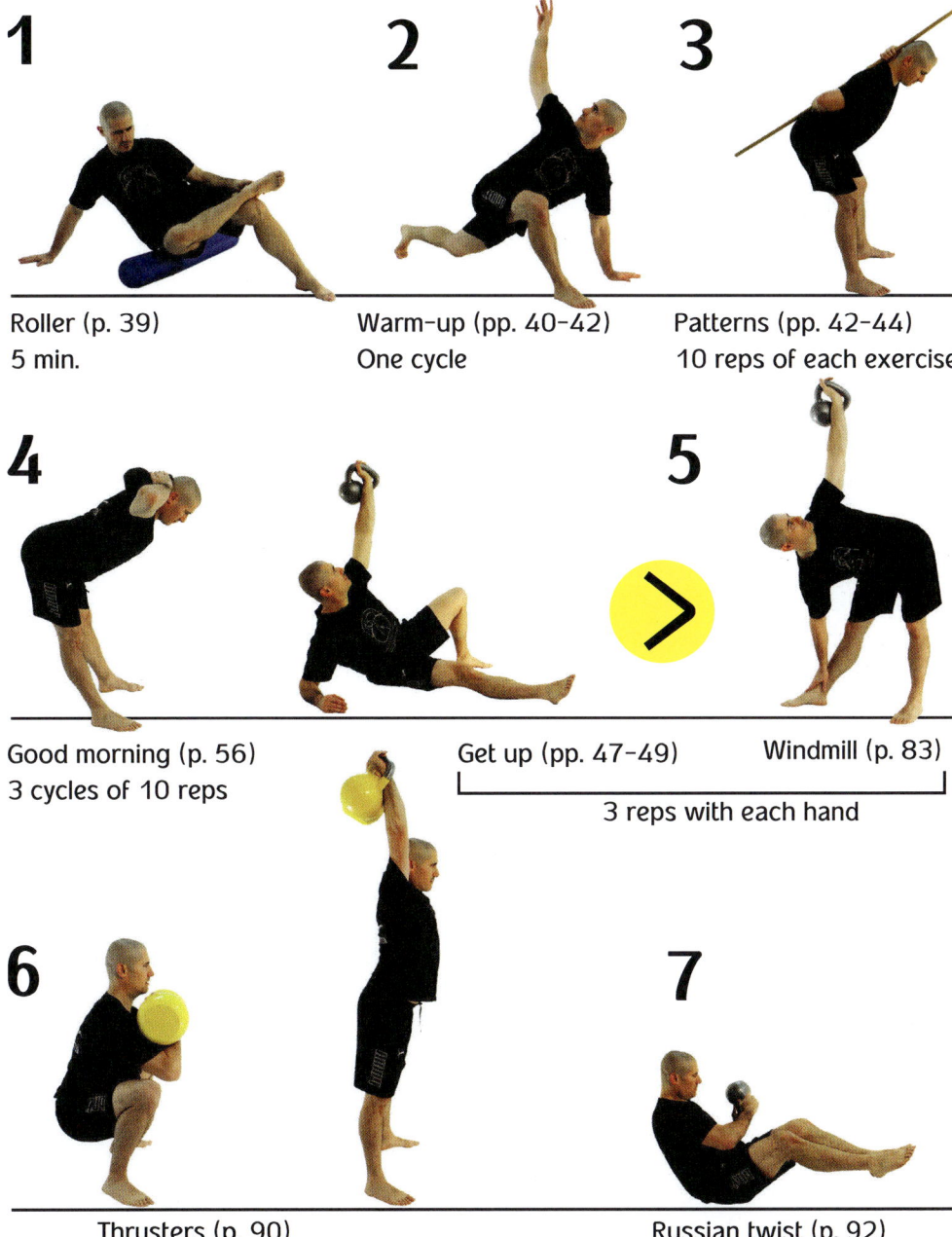

1

Roller (p. 39)
5 min.

2

Warm-up (pp. 40-42)
One cycle

3

Patterns (pp. 42-44)
10 reps of each exercise

4

Good morning (p. 56)
3 cycles of 10 reps

5

Get up (pp. 47-49)   Windmill (p. 83)

3 reps with each hand

6

Thrusters (p. 90)
2 cycles of 10 repetitions

7

Russian twist (p. 92)
2 cycles of 20 repetitions

6.1.5 30-minute practice program

The program is intended for independent daily practice.
The practice is suitable for exercisers at all levels who have had basic instruction.

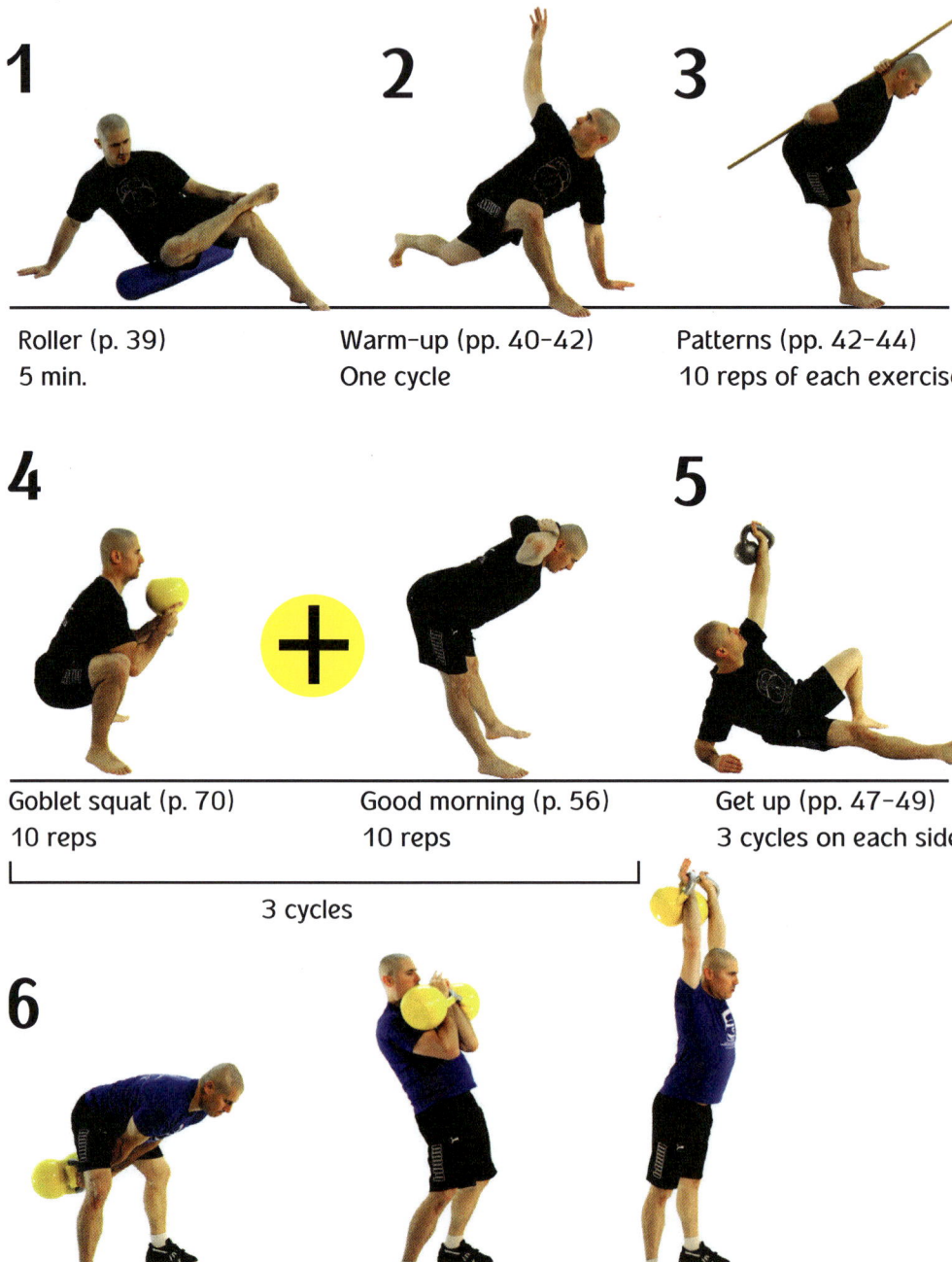

1 Roller (p. 39)
5 min.

2 Warm-up (pp. 40–42)
One cycle

3 Patterns (pp. 42–44)
10 reps of each exercise

4 Goblet squat (p. 70)
10 reps

+ Good morning (p. 56)
10 reps

5 Get up (pp. 47–49)
3 cycles on each side

3 cycles

6 Long cycle (pp. 78–80) 3 cycles of 3 minutes

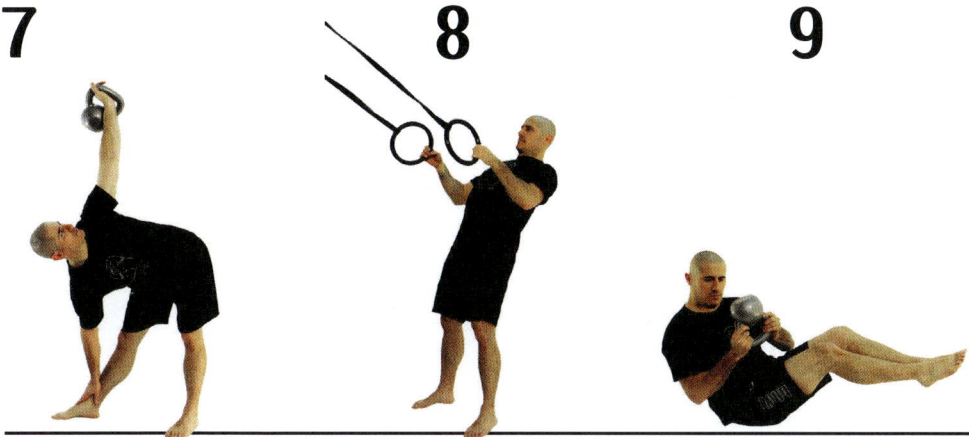

7

8

9

Windmill (p. 83)
2 cycles of 5 reps
for each hand

Pull up / Ring pull (p. 96)
2 cycles of 20 reps

Russian twist (p. 92)
2 cycles of 20 repetitions

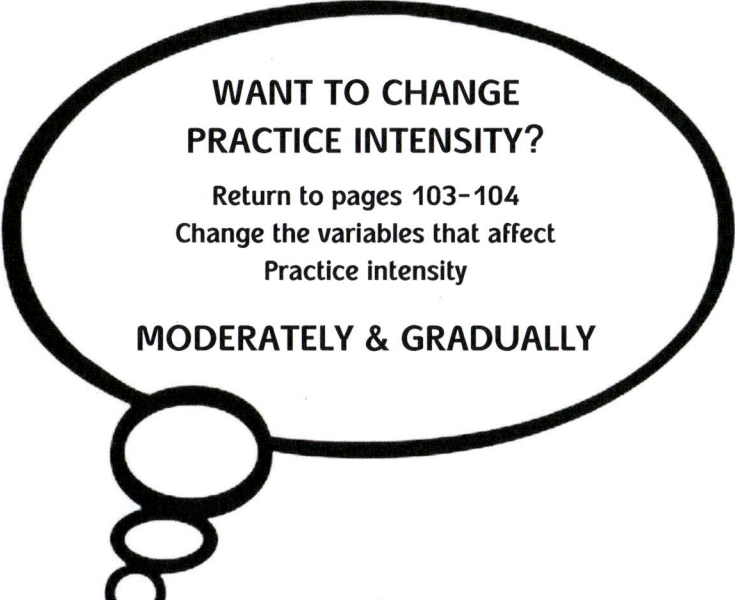

WANT TO CHANGE
PRACTICE INTENSITY?

**Return to pages 103-104
Change the variables that affect
Practice intensity**

MODERATELY & GRADUALLY

6.1.6 30-minute practice program

The program is intended for independent daily practice.
The practice is suitable for exercisers at all levels who have had basic instruction.

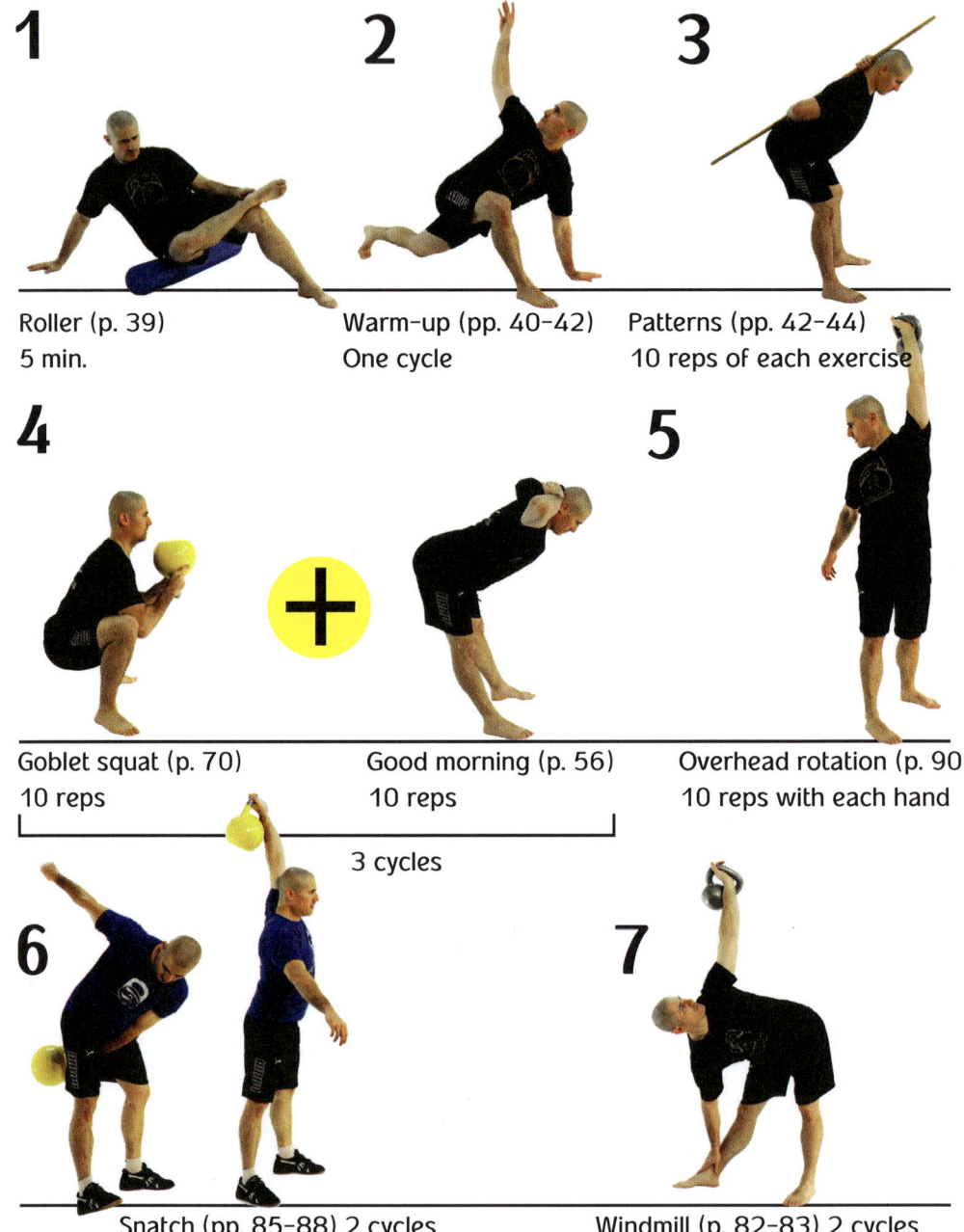

1

Roller (p. 39)
5 min.

2

Warm-up (pp. 40–42)
One cycle

3

Patterns (pp. 42–44)
10 reps of each exercise

4

Goblet squat (p. 70)
10 reps

+

Good morning (p. 56)
10 reps

5

Overhead rotation (p. 90)
10 reps with each hand

3 cycles

6

Snatch (pp. 85–88) 2 cycles
of 2 minutes per hand

7

Windmill (p. 82–83) 2 cycles
of 5 reps per hand

8

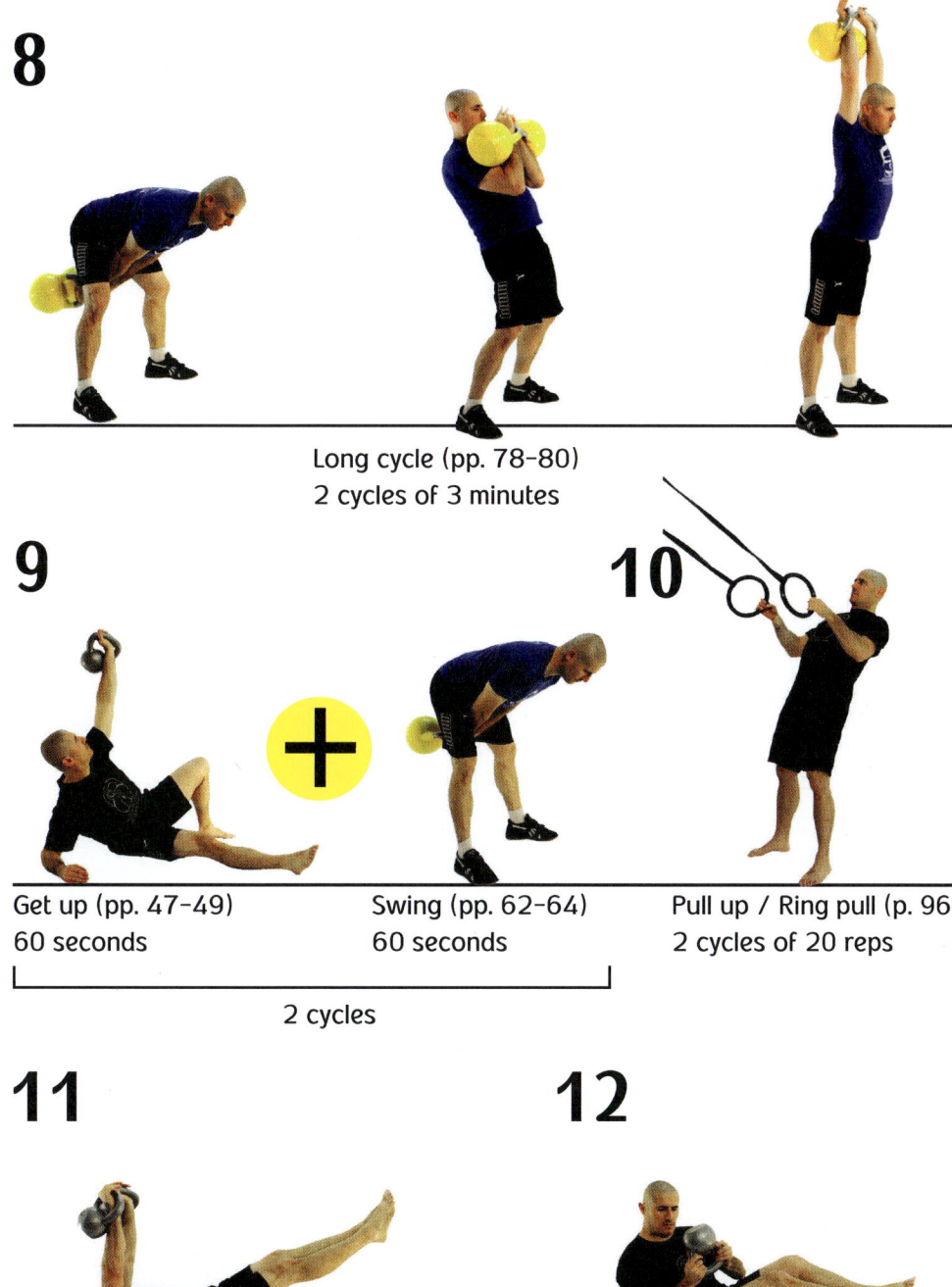

Long cycle (pp. 78–80)
2 cycles of 3 minutes

9

10

Get up (pp. 47–49)
60 seconds

Swing (pp. 62–64)
60 seconds

Pull up / Ring pull (p. 96)
2 cycles of 20 reps

2 cycles

11

12

Leg lift (p. 93)
2 cycles of 20 reps

Russian twist (p. 92)
2 cycles of 20 repetitions

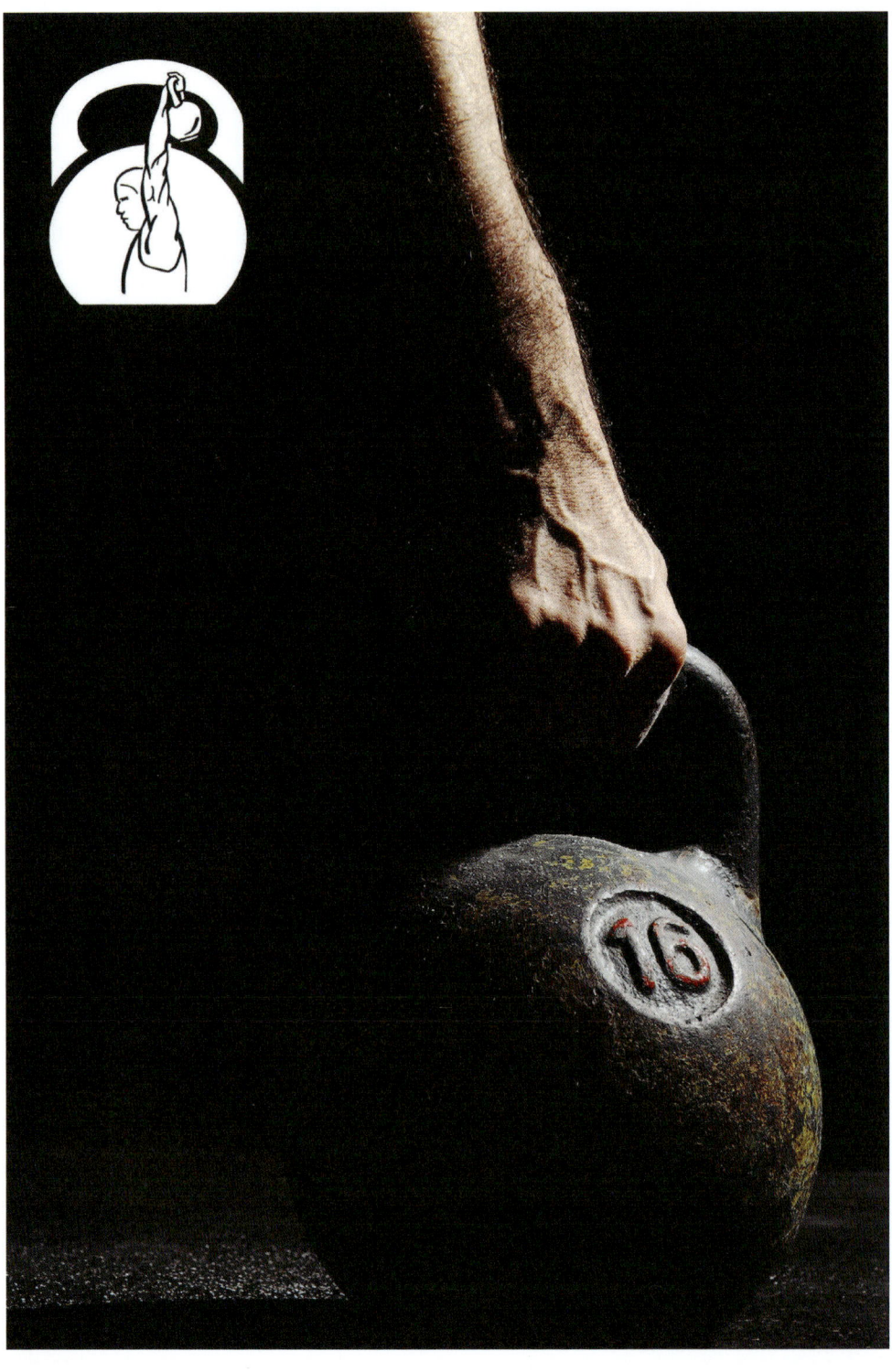

CHAPTER 7

USEFUL INFORMATION

- Lists of instructors and clubs in Israel

- Kettlebells roots workshop

- Kettlebell Instructors Course

- Guide for Acquiring Kettlebells

7. USEFUL INFORMATION

For lists of instructors, kettlebell workshops, instructors' training courses and professional information:
www.kettlebells.co.il

For additional questions and information send an email to: hirschuri@gmail.com

7.1 Lists of instructors and clubs in Israel
Want to swing? Choose a certified instructor from the Israel Kettlebells Association!
The list of kettlebell instructors of the Israel Kettlebells Association can be found at:
www.kettlebells.co.il
Main club: Eitanim Kettlebells - 50 Rabbi Akiva St. Herzlia, Israel

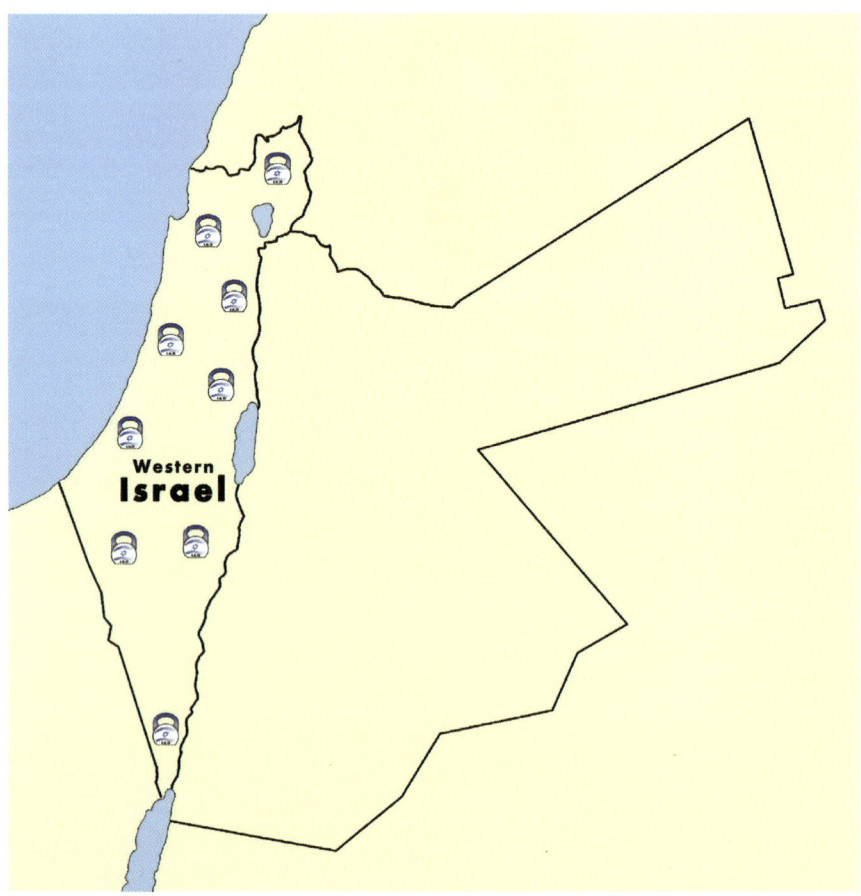

7.2 Kettlebells Roots Workshop

For coaches, instructors and exercisers, sponsored by the Israel Kettlebells Association.

Aims of the workshop:

- To learn what functional movement practice is and the logic behind kettlebell practice
- To impart basic personal information for the safe and effective use of kettlebells
- Practical tools for functional movement practice
- The structure and uniqueness of kettlebells
- Learning and practicing: dead lift, get-up and tailoring exercises to the exerciser's physique
- And other secrets that no one has ever told you about kettlebells....

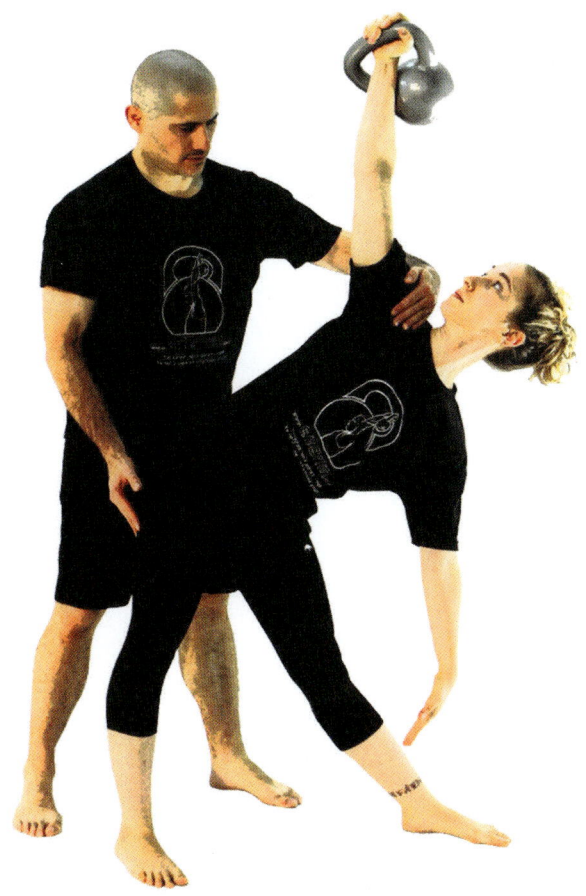

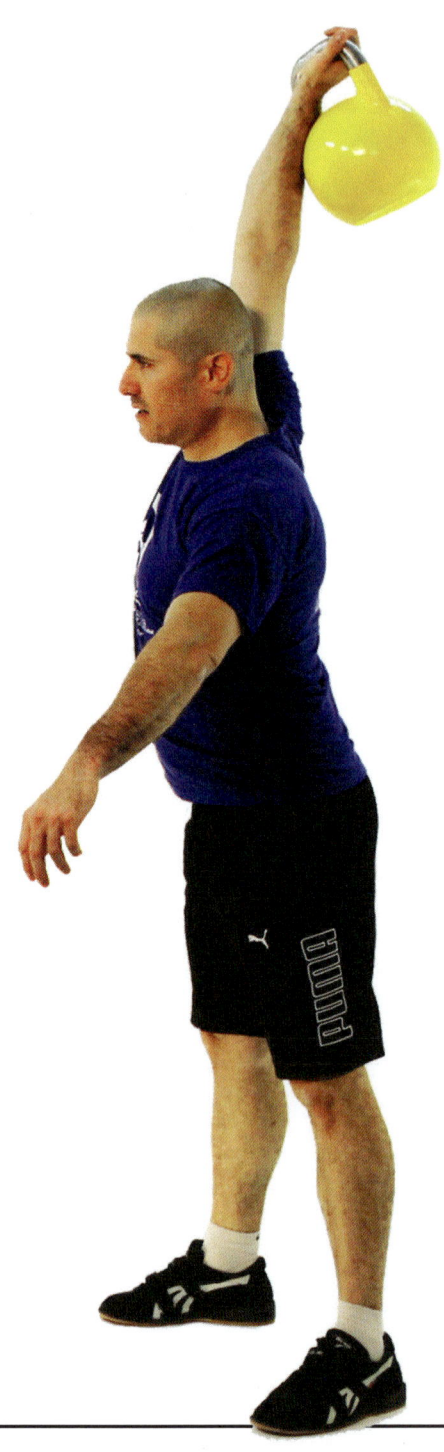

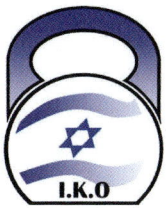 

7.3 Kettlebells Instructors Course

Functional movement practice using kettlebells - for conducting group lessons and personal training. Given by the Israel Kettlebells Association.

Course aims:

- To train kettlebell instructors for group lessons and personal training
- To learn and understand the theory of functional movement practice and its practical implementation using kettlebells
- Teaching methods: Lectures with demonstrations and learning through movement
- The course curriculum for training kettlebells instructors meets international standards and offers a wide variety of unique professional material taught clearly and understandably.

Target population

Fitness and health instructors, physical education teachers, teachers of the martial arts, studio instructors for body sculpting, aerobics, yoga, Pilates, posture and dance who wish to upgrade their professional qualifications, enrich their professional knowledge, learn about body mobility, and add depth, ideas and exercises to training. The course is suitable for instructors who have completed other kettlebell training and exercisers who are interested in increasing their familiarity with functioning training with kettlebells.

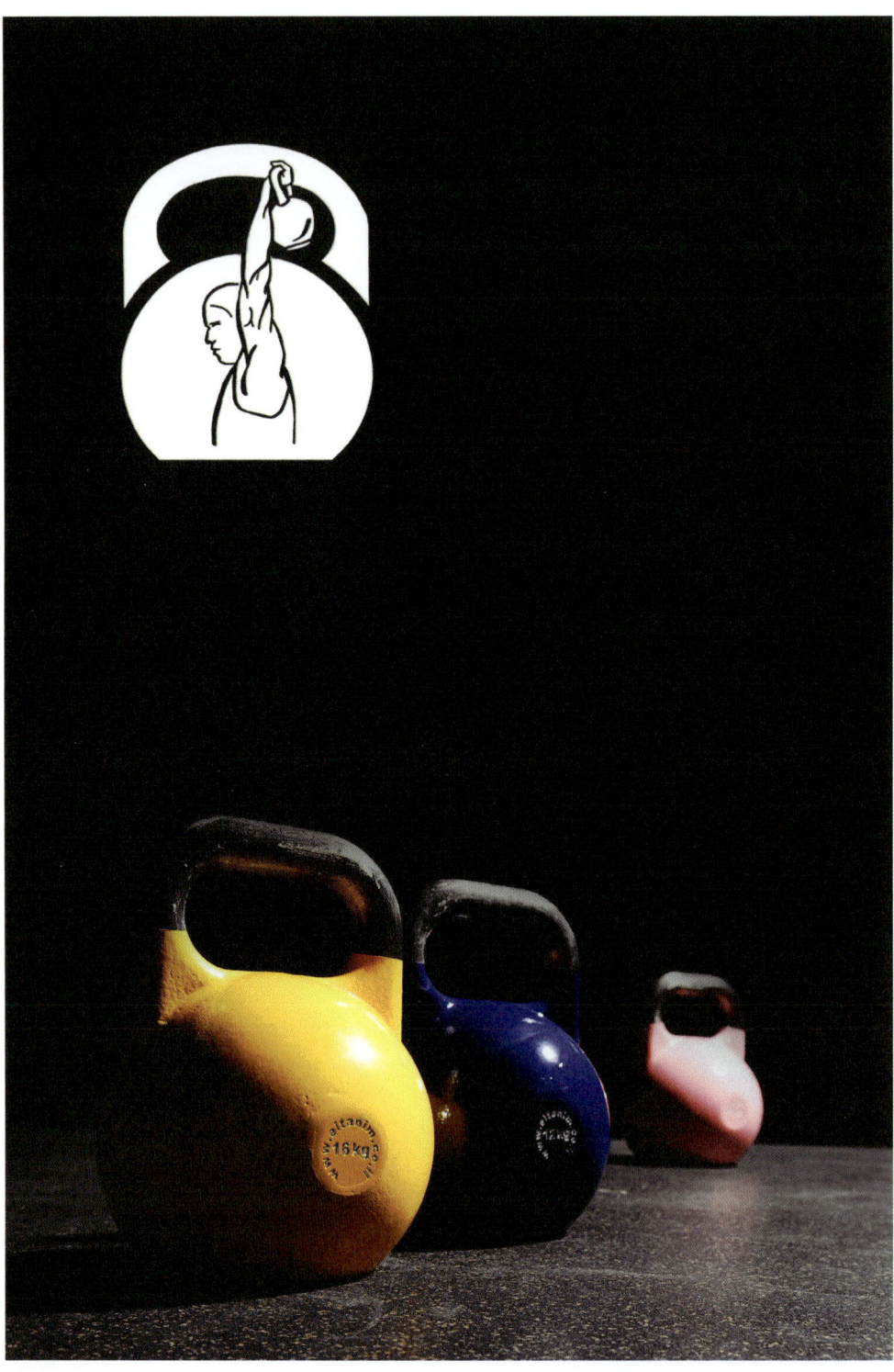

7.4 The guide to acquiring kettlebells

Differences between classic kettlebells and competitive kettlebells

Classic kettlebells

Handle thickness and kettlebell size vary according to weight. In other words, a 4 kg kettlebell will be smaller than a 48 kg kettlebell.
- Made of cast iron
- More comfortable for women and people with a small physique. More comfortable for exercises like Windmill and Get up.
- Color – black
- Suitable for fitness instructors, personal trainers, crossfit and exercisers who are not expert in kettlebells.

Competitive kettlebells

Handle thickness and kettlebell size are the same for all weights. This uniformity of handle thickness and size has a number of advantages for competitive kettlebells:
- The swing technique remains the same in each weight. In other words, as the load is gradually increased, the body learns to move in the same way and with accurate technique whether the kettlebell is heavier or lighter.
- The kettlebell structure and handle are more comfortable for swing exercises and the long exercise.
- Kettlebell colors: 8kg – pink, 12 – blue, 16 – yellow, 20 – purple, 24 – green, 28 – orange, 32 – red, 36 – grey, 40 – white, 44 – silver, 48 – gold.
- Used by kettlebell exercisers and coaches in the sport style.

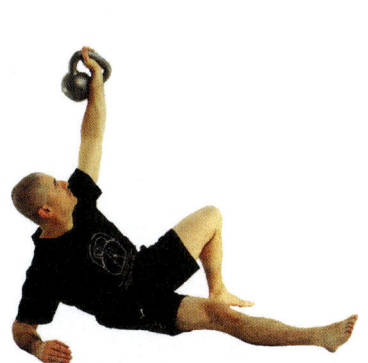

Classic kettlebell

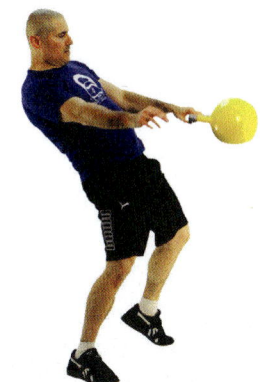

Competitive kettlebell

What is the best weight kettlebell to start with?

To determine the best weight to begin with, a number of variables should be considered:
- Exerciser's state of physical fitness
- Movement ability
- Health status (limitations, posture, etc.)
- Gender
- Age

Weight recommendations for initial purchase

Ability		Male	Female
Low	No training background; after injury; small physique	8-12 kg	4-8 kg
Medium	Training background; good movement ability; medium physique	12-16 kg	8-12 kg
High	Athletic, strong, large physique	16-24 kg	12-16 kg

Eitanim Kettlebells (1964)
Importers and marketers of professional equipment
for movement practice and functional fitness
www.functionaltraining.co.il

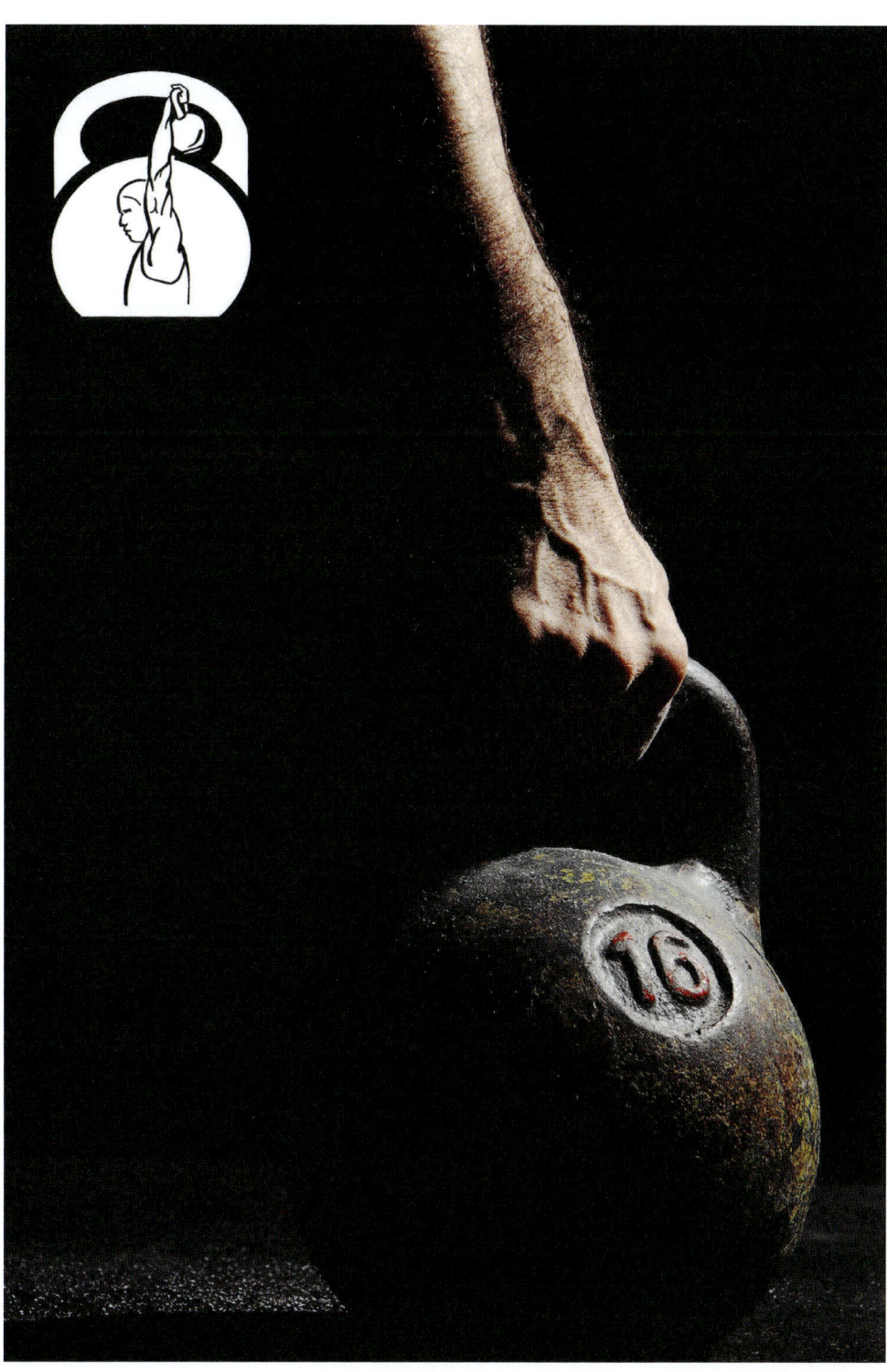

Note on the Land of Israel map (p. 120)

The map of Israel on page 120 is based on the League of Nations document "The Mandate for Palestine" (1923), which details the legal rights of the Jewish people in Palestine*.
The Council of the League of Nations:
"Whereas the Principal Allied Powers have also agreed that the Mandatory should be responsible for putting into effect the declaration originally made on November 2nd, 1917, by the Government of His Britannic Majesty, and adopted by the said Powers, in favor of the establishment in Palestine of a national home for the Jewish people, ... Whereas recognition has thereby been given to the historical connection of the Jewish people with Palestine and to the grounds for reconstituting their national home in that country;" (Mandate for Palestine - 1923)

US Under-Secretary of Defense Douglas Feith: "The argument that the Jews have no legal right to settle in Samaria and Judea tends inevitably, even if unintentionally, to undermine the Jewish people's right to sovereignty in pre-1967 Israel, for all such rights flow from the same source - the Palestine Mandate recognizing the Jewish people's historical connection with Palestine."

Levy Commission Report (Honorable Supreme Court Judge (Ret.) Edmond Levy, Honorable Judge Tchiya Shapiro and attorney Alan Baker, an expert on international law: "From the point of view of International law, Israelis have the lawful right to settle in Judea and Samaria"
*Palestine was the English name used to describe the Land of Israel (national home for the Jewish people) until 1947.

Printed in Great Britain
by Amazon